Emerging Issues in Family and Individual Resilience

Series Editors
Amanda W. Harrist
Stephan M. Wilson

More information about this series at http://www.springer.com/series/13415

Whitney A. Bailey • Amanda W. Harrist
Editors

Family Caregiving

Fostering Resilience Across the Life Course

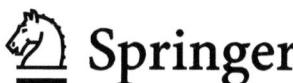

Editors
Whitney A. Bailey
Oklahoma State University
Stillwater, OK, USA

Amanda W. Harrist
Oklahoma State University
Stillwater, OK, USA

ISSN 2366-6072   ISSN 2366-6080 (electronic)
Emerging Issues in Family and Individual Resilience
ISBN 978-3-319-64782-1   ISBN 978-3-319-64783-8 (eBook)
DOI 10.1007/978-3-319-64783-8

Library of Congress Control Number: 2017953391

© Springer International Publishing AG 2018
This work is subject to copyright. All rights are reserved by the Publisher, whether the whole or part of the material is concerned, specifically the rights of translation, reprinting, reuse of illustrations, recitation, broadcasting, reproduction on microfilms or in any other physical way, and transmission or information storage and retrieval, electronic adaptation, computer software, or by similar or dissimilar methodology now known or hereafter developed.
The use of general descriptive names, registered names, trademarks, service marks, etc. in this publication does not imply, even in the absence of a specific statement, that such names are exempt from the relevant protective laws and regulations and therefore free for general use.
The publisher, the authors and the editors are safe to assume that the advice and information in this book are believed to be true and accurate at the date of publication. Neither the publisher nor the authors or the editors give a warranty, express or implied, with respect to the material contained herein or for any errors or omissions that may have been made. The publisher remains neutral with regard to jurisdictional claims in published maps and institutional affiliations.

Printed on acid-free paper

This Springer imprint is published by Springer Nature
The registered company is Springer International Publishing AG
The registered company address is: Gewerbestrasse 11, 6330 Cham, Switzerland

Preface

It is projected that those 65 years and older will comprise 20% of the US population by the year 2030, with the fastest growing segment being those 85+ years (CDC, *The State of Aging and Health in America 2013*). Approximately 92% of older adults have at least one chronic disease, and 77% have at least two (NCOA, 2017). While medical technology can enable us to live longer, it does not protect us from associated illnesses such as cancer, cardiovascular disease, and musculoskeletal disease. The experience of exceptional longevity (i.e., living >100 years) is increasingly common. Yet, quality of life is not maintained. *While the demographic research is informative and vast, it is not enough to simply know we are living longer with greater likelihood of diseases.*

Providing care for one another has been at the heart of family functioning since the beginning of time. From an early age, individuals are socialized to interact with one another based on social rules, cultural norms, developmental expectations, and family meaning. Governmental rules and policies are central to the ways family and kin members function in helping one another. A key element to the ways in which state and federal policies shape caregiving in the Unites States includes "the Caregiver Assumption" (Bailey & Gordon, 2016). This refers to the expectation that a family will care for its members during acute and chronic health challenges. This is magnified by a system that prioritizes home and community-based services (HCBS) over institutionalized care. On the surface, this value—keeping people at home as long as possible—is shared by governmental systems and families alike. Yet, implementation of HCBS is done at the expense of family and kin caregivers, their health, financial futures, and other relationships. Because of the way we do caregiving in the United States, caregivers are at greater risk for providing care well beyond the scope of their abilities, increasing risk of injury (to themselves or their loved ones), which then perpetuates the cycle of risk and need for care. Family caregiving is truly a public health crisis, not only because it is inherently demanding but because of the *way* we provide care. Consequently, service and support of elders and their family caregivers is a critical public health issue. *We have known the challenges for decades, yet it is not enough to know the challenges.*

This volume seeks to provide those in the human sciences and related fields a base of topical chapters related to the caregiving experience. Resilience as a process and an outcome is a common theme throughout. Each chapter identifies the risks present in caregiving situations, while offering tips and resources for care families. So often, care families do not know where to start. The National Alliance for Caregiving and AARP's Public Policy study (2015) revealed that 84% of caregivers need more information and training to care for their loved ones. Simultaneously, many professionals do not feel equipped to assist because, with rare exception, the primary and higher education systems have failed to prepare the workforce to serve this burgeoning need. It's not as if we didn't see it coming. Yet, this volume was born out of the belief that even professionals who do not identify with the field of "Gerontology" or "Aging Studies" have the opportunity to help care families. After all, with 84% of caregivers reporting a need for more information and training in their care roles, surely each person who is reading this can do something to fill that gap. *It is not enough to say "it isn't my area."*

The opportunity now lies with us to address this public health crisis, utilizing the family resilience framework as a guide. With the passage of the CARE Act in more than 20 states, elected officials and the aging network are showing signs that they are mobilizing and primed for change in this area. Our opportunity lies in knowing what shapes caregiving experiences in our respective states and then responding: through education, advocacy, engagement, intervention, or any domain for that matter. Whether you are an advocate, researcher, educator, or practitioner, there is a need to improve the ways caregivers understand the system, access the system, and do the business of caregiving. Countless studies have shown us the risks of providing care, with little focus on protective processes. Utilizing the resilience model allows us to change the perspective from one of disadvantage and hardship to a strengths-based approach. Eighty-four percent of caregivers report needing more information and training in their care roles (2015). *We know enough to know the need. We know enough to know the consequences are life changing. Find your sphere of influence and go!*

Stillwater, OK, USA   Whitney A. Bailey
                                                                              Kristopher M. Struckmeyer

References

Bailey, W. A. & Gordon, S. R. (2016). Family caregiving amidst age-associated cognitive changes: Implications for practice and future generations. *Family Relations,* (65). doi:10.1111/fare.12176

Caregiving in the U.S. (June, 2015). AARP Public Policy Institute and the National Alliance on Caregiving: Washington, D.C.

National Council on Aging. (2017). News for reporters. Retrieved from https://www.ncoa.org/news/resources-for-reporters/get-the-facts/healthy-aging-facts/

The State of Aging and Health in America 2013. Centers for Disease Control and Prevention, US Department of Health and Human Services: Atlanta, GA.

Acknowledgements

Oklahoma State University's Center for Family Resilience (CFR) hosts an annual *Chautauqua: Conference on Family Resilience*. The goals of the conference are (a) to bring together distinguished and rising scholars from diverse disciplines to discuss cutting-edge work focused on one annual theme within the broader area of family resilience research, and (b) to foster a translational approach within the study of resilience, such that practical applications for family health and well-being can be developed from basic resilience research. This includes development of action steps in conjunction with community stakeholders. The papers presented at each year's Chautauqua are the core of the chapters that comprise the respective volume in our *Emerging Issues in Family and Individual Resilience* series. We would like to thank the many people involved in planning and hosting the 2016 Chautauqua. These include OSU Human Development and Family Science (HDFS) doctoral students Zach Giano, Amy Huffer, Rebecca Hubbard, Ashley Kimble, Todd Spencer, Erin Seseman, Julie Staton, and Brooke Tuttle, who helped facilitate the Chautauqua discussion sessions and host the authors' dinner, and Kris Struckmeyer, who coordinated transportation; HDFS staff, especially Rita Ryan, who coordinated financial issues; and Dr. Christine Johnson, Lisa Smith, and Tia Claybrook, who helped with the many details of conference planning and implementation.

We are extremely grateful to those who helped fund the 2016 Chautauqua that made this volume possible. Thank you to Dr. Michael Merten for providing funding from the CFR and Dr. Whitney Bailey for funds from the Bryan Close Professorship in Adulthood and Aging. Special thanks to AARP Oklahoma, who was instrumental in supporting the authors' event that helped formulate this volume. We thank AARP Oklahoma for their sponsorship and applaud their leadership and advocacy for what became the nation's first CARE Act in 2014.

For the preparation of this volume, we are indebted to editors Jennifer Hadley and Sara Yanny-Tillar at Springer, who were so helpful and patient with us, despite the fact that it took longer to "birth" this book than it did to bring Baby Max into the world! Thank you also to CFR Research Associates Dr. Ron Cox, Dr. Greg Clare, Dr. Catherine Curtis, Sally Eagleton, Dr. Kami Gallus, Chelsea Keel, Dr. Robert Larzelere, Dr. Amanda Morris, Canada Parrish, and Dr. Martha Roblyer, who reviewed and edited the volume's chapters; they also conducted interviews and wrote the breakout boxes appearing in each chapter of Volume 2 and we are grateful for that. Finally, we are indebted to the community professionals and families who were willing to contribute to the breakout boxes that provide practical application and advice to professionals in each chapter.

We also acknowledge and are appreciative of the many resilient caregivers in our community and worldwide who give their time and love to family members in need every day. We dedicate this volume to them.

About the Series Editors

Amanda W. Harrist received her Ph.D. in Child and Family Studies from the University of Tennessee, Knoxville. She is currently a Professor of Human Development and Family Science at Oklahoma State University, where she is also Associate Director for Education and Translation at the Center for Family Resilience and Core Director, Human & Community Research Training Core for the Center for Integrative Research on Childhood Adversity. Her research is focused on understanding psychosocial risk and protective processes in children's social contexts, particularly the parent-child relationship and peer relations at school.

Stephan M. Wilson is a Ph.D. graduate in Child and Family Studies from the University of Tennessee, Knoxville. He is an NCFR Fellow, Fulbright Fellow, Regents Professor at Oklahoma State University, Legend recognition of the American Association of Family and Consumer Sciences, and has numerous teaching, research, and community engagement recognitions. His areas of expertise include cross-cultural family science and adolescent social competence.

Contents

1 **Family Resilience and Caregiving** 1
   Carolyn S. Henry, Rebecca L. Hubbard, Kristopher M. Struckmeyer,
   and Todd A. Spencer

2 **Therapeutic Interventions for Caregiving Families** 27
   Sara Honn Qualls

3 **Resilience Through Nutrition: Nutritional and Dietary
   Challenges and Opportunities for Caregiving Families** 45
   Janice R. Hermann and Kristopher M. Struckmeyer

4 **Caregiver Resilience: Improving Ergonomics for the Safety,
   Comfort, and Health of Caregivers** 63
   Aditya Jayadas and Mihyun Kang

5 **Hope as a Coping Resource for Caregiver Resilience
   and Well-Being** 81
   Chan M. Hellman, Jody A. Worley, and Ricky T. Munoz

6 **Voices from Down Home: Family Caregiver Perspectives
   on Navigating Care Transitions with Individuals
   with Dementia in Nova Scotia, Canada** 99
   Emily Roberts

7 **Planning for and Managing Costs Related to Caregiving** 121
   Louise A. Schroeder and Sissy R. Osteen

Index 143

Contributors

Chan M. Hellman, Ph.D. College of Arts and Sciences, University of Oklahoma, Tulsa and OU Center of Applied Research for Nonprofit Organizations, Tulsa, OK, USA

Carolyn S. Henry, Ph.D. Department of Human Development and Family Science, Oklahoma State University, Stillwater, OK, USA

Janice R. Hermann, Ph.D., R.D./L.D Department of Nutritional Sciences, Oklahoma State University, Stillwater, OK, USA

Rebecca L. Hubbard Department of Human Development and Family Science, Oklahoma State University, Tulsa, OK, USA

Aditya Jayadas, Ph.D. Department of Design Housing and Merchandising, Oklahoma State University, Stillwater, OK, USA

Mihyun Kang, Ph.D. Department of Design Housing and Merchandising, Oklahoma State University, Stillwater, OK, USA

Ricky T. Munoz, J.D. Anne and Henry Zarrow School of Social Work and OU Center of Applied Research for Nonprofit Organizations, Tulsa, OK, USA

Sissy R. Osteen, Ph.D., CFP® Human Development and Family Science, Oklahoma State University, Stillwater, OK, USA

Sara Honn Qualls, Ph.D. University of Colorado Colorado Springs, Psychology Department and Gerontology Center, Colorado Springs, CO, USA

Emily Roberts, Ph.D. Department of Design, Housing, and Merchandising, College of Human Sciences, Oklahoma, Oklahoma State University, Stillwater, OK, USA

Louise A. Schroeder, CFP® Certified Financial Planner™ Professional, Stillwater, OK, USA

Todd A. Spencer Department of Human Development and Family Science, Oklahoma State University, Stillwater, OK, USA

Kristopher M. Struckmeyer Department of Human Development and Family Science, Oklahoma State University, Stillwater, OK, USA

Jody A. Worley, Ph.D. OU Department of Human Relations and Center of Applied Research for Nonprofit Organizations, Tulsa, OK, USA

Chapter 1
Family Resilience and Caregiving

Carolyn S. Henry, Rebecca L. Hubbard, Kristopher M. Struckmeyer, and Todd A. Spencer

Family caregiving occurs as one or more family members provide care to at least one other family member defined by the family or professionals as requiring assistance in at least one key domain of life (Walker, Pratt, & Eddy, 1995). Over time, caregiving occurs in most families as challenges in one or more areas of well-being such as physical, cognitive, or emotional well-being. In addition, caregivers often become informal case managers who coordinate care across multiple settings and providers, maintain interpersonal contact and advocacy with multiple care providers. Family members may gradually drift into, actively choose, or quickly accept caregiving during a crisis (Bailey & Gordon, 2016; Johnston, Bailey, & Wilson, 2014; Qualls & Williams, 2013). As demands increase through the daily hassles and new responsibilities of caregiving, on-going family relationship patterns require change, often involving more frequent and intense family interfaces with proximal (or close) ecosystems including medical and social services (see Table 1.1). We use the terminology of "care recipient" for individuals receiving care and "caregiver" for individuals caring for care recipients, recognizing that both caregivers and care recipients have a sense of self and family beyond these roles. In fact, individuals can be mutual caregivers and care recipients such as when spouses provide care to each other. Caregiving burden arises through ongoing daily hassles, difficult decisions, sacrifices, and other demands that increase the risk for stress, burnout, and declines in caregivers' health, self-care, and the ability to fulfill other life roles (Zarit, Reever, & Bach-Peterson, 1980). The unique combination of caregiver burden in specific

---

C.S. Henry, Ph.D. (✉) • K.M. Struckmeyer, M.S. • T.A. Spencer, M.S.
Department of Human Development and Family Science, Oklahoma State University, Stillwater, OK 74078-6122, USA
e-mail: carolyn.henry@okstate.edu; struckm@okstate.edu; todd.spencer@okstate.edu

R.L. Hubbard, M.S.
Department of Human Development and Family Science, Oklahoma State University, 700 N. Greenwood, Tulsa, OK 74016, USA
e-mail: rebecca.hubbard@okstate.edu

Table 1.1 Progression of dementia: challenges for care recipients, caregivers, family adaptive systems, and family-ecosystem interface

	Stage of dementia			
	Mild disease progression	Moderate disease progression	Severe disease progression	Nearing death and grief
Challenges for care recipients	Loss of words	Unable to do simple math	Significant confusion	Loss of ability to respond to others (loss smile, eye contact, holding head up, speech)
	Forget names	Forgets some life history details	Behavior problems	Loss of ability to interact with environment
	Difficulty planning or organizing	Decreased ability in short term memory	Loss of speech	Needs help with all ADLs
	Begin short term memory loss	Difficulty managing finances or paying bills	Significant personality changes	Loss of bodily functions (possibly including the ability to swallow)
		Progressing to	Unable to recognize faces	
		Significant confusion	Needs significant help with ADLs	
		Difficulty in recall of simple information (e.g. their phone number)	Cannot remember most of personal history	
		Difficulty dressing weather appropriate	Loss of bowel and bladder control	
			Difficulty expressing needs	

1 Family Resilience and Caregiving

Challenges for caregivers	Balancing help with autonomy	Balancing help with autonomy	Balancing help with autonomy	Understanding and accepting imminent decline and death process
	Understanding the diagnosis	Understanding the diagnosis	Understanding the progression of the disease	Preparing for death transition
	Adapting to changes and partner's decline in mental abilities	Understanding progression of the disease	Adapting to changes and partner's mental and physical decline	Coordinating care and family or ecosystem assistance
	Begin assisting and taking over financial responsibilities for care recipient	Taking over previously held responsibilities of care recipient	Adjusting to changes in relationship	
		Adapting to changes and partner's decline in mental abilities	Coordinating care and family or ecosystem assistance	
		Adjusting to changes in relationship		
		Coordinating care and family or ecosystem assistance		
Challenges for family adaptive systems	Potential changes in FES and FMS	Potential challenges in FES, FMS, FCS, and FMNS[a]	Likely challenges in FCS and FMNS	Likely challenges in FCS, FMS, FES, and FMNS
			Potential challenges in FES and FMS	

(continued)

Table 1.1 (continued)

	Stage of dementia			
	Mild disease progression	Moderate disease progression	Severe disease progression	Nearing death and grief
Challenges for family-ecosystem interface	Medical care	Medical care	Medical care	Medical care
		Social system support	Social services	Social system support
			Social system support	Ancillary services
			Ancillary services	Hospice

Notes: Families involved in caregiving for family members with dementia share the experience of progression of the condition according to individual pathways that are somewhat predictable, yet highly individualized in timing and intensity. The progression of dementia symptoms is progressive in the overall trajectory (National Institute of Health, 2016)

[a]The five stages in this model are based on coalescing existing stages of dementia (Alzheimer's Association, 2016; Alzheimer's Society, 2016; Morris, 1993; National Institute on Aging, 2016; Reisberg, 1988) that range from three to seven stages. This composite model describes challenges for care recipients, caregivers, family adaptive systems, and family-ecosystem interfaces. This guide shows general trends in progression whereas in reality, each person with dementia progresses through individualized stages

[b]*FES family emotion system, FMS family meaning system, FCS family control system, FMNS family maintenance system*

families at specific points in time involves not only care recipient and caregiver needs, but also family dynamics, family perceptions of the situation, and other co-occurring stressors. Although family caregiving spans the life course, we focus on caregiving of adult members. Building on these ideas, we present the Family Resilience Model (Henry, Morris, & Harrist, 2015) as a framework for policy makers, researchers, and practitioners to understand how individuals, subsystems, overall family systems, and families-proximal ecosystem relationships interface in caregiving.

1.1 Family Caregiving Through the Lens of the Family Resilience Model

We share a modification of the Family Resilience Model (FRM; Henry et al., 2015, Fig. 1.1) (see Fig. 1.2) as a promising approach to understanding how families can address caregiving and other demands in ways that allow them to function as well as or better than before caregiving began. Caregiving intertwines with family system dynamics such that stress in one part of a family system reverberates throughout the system (Qualls, this volume; Qualls & Williams, 2013). Two modifications of the FRM are included in Fig. 1.2, (a) listing the multiple levels of family systems and (b) distinguishing between proximal and distal ecosystems (see Fig. 1.2). Family caregiving involves multiple family systems levels: each individual family member (e.g., care recipient, caregiver, adult children, grandchildren), family

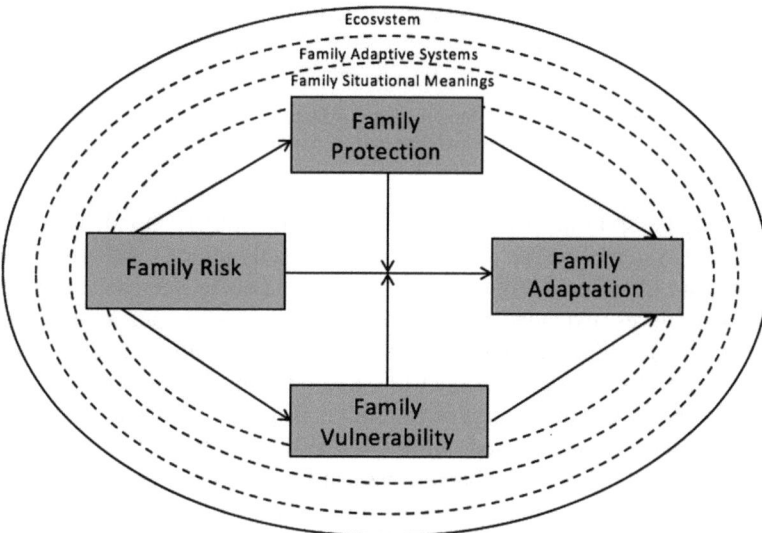

Fig. 1.1 Family Resilience Model (Permission to reprint this figure from Henry et al., 2015 granted by John Wiley & Sons)

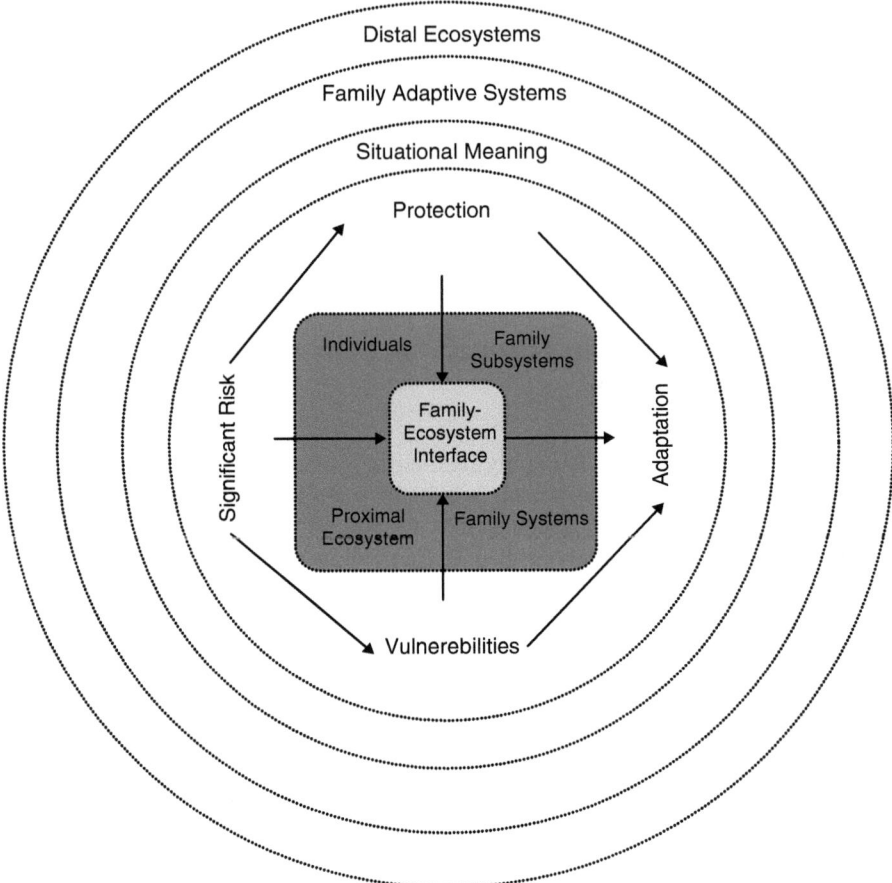

Fig. 1.2 Modified Family Resilience Model. *Note*: Adapted from the Family Resilience Model (Henry et al., 2015) to illustrate system levels and to distinguish proximal and distal ecosystems

subsystems (e.g., spousal, parent-child, sibling, grandparent-grandchild), and the overall family system (see Fig. 1.2). Caregivers directly interact with proximal ecosystems of care often including multiple medical and social service care providers, schools, workplaces, extended family systems, religious organizations, insurance and other financial organizations as well as other systems (Moon, 2017). Caregiving occurs with distal ecosystems critical to caregiving involve policies and funding regulated by systems that are part of the social structure governing health care or social/aging services, and related entities, as well as culture (Taylor & Quesnel-Vallée, 2017). Throughout the chapter, we use family members with dementia to illustrate key points, providing a case study of a caregiving family with a member with dementia.

1.1.1 Core Concepts

We begin by discussing five core resilience concepts integrated into the FRM—significant risk, protection, vulnerability, adaptation, and family situational meanings—followed by family and ecosystem concepts that are critical to understanding resilience in families engaged in caregiving (see Fig. 1.2).

1.1.1.1 Significant Risk

Significant risk is necessary for resilience to occur (Wright, Masten, & Narayan, 2013). *Significant risk* occurs when families perceive an imbalance between their capabilities and demands, threatening the short- or long- term functioning in one or more parts of their family system (Patterson, 2002). Family caregiving is a significant risk, both through status risk and specific stressor events (see Qualls & Williams, 2013; Walsh, 2012b). First, caregiving *status risk* is present as families live with the vertical (or on-going) challenges associated with providing care for family members (McGoldrick & Shibusawa, 2012). The focus on the caregiving needs of one family member, for example, might disrupt ongoing rules, roles, and interactions in family systems such that needs of one or more other family members and/or the family system are neglected (Cornille & Boroto, 1992). The extent of caregiver burden varies over time with the ebb and flow of care needs over time often pile-up and may intensify over time (Haley, 2003; Zarit et al., 1980). Although caregiver burden is often applied to individuals who are caregivers, caregiver burden also occurs in family systems as care demands create stress by disrupting ongoing dynamics of the overall family system, In turn, each time caregiving demands shift, on-going family interaction patterns require rebalancing.

Significant caregiving risk also arises through *specific family stressors* at specific times when families perceive their current demands to outweigh their social, psychological, or material capabilities (Patterson, 2002). Such stressors, known as horizontal stressors, occur over time through historic events, family life cycle transitions (e.g., birth of a grandchild, adolescent transitioning out of high school, retirement), the hospitalization of a care recipient, or changes in the care needs (e.g., change in a caregiver's condition) (McGoldrick & Shibusawa, 2012). The progression of degenerative health conditions (e.g., Alzheimer's disease) (Komarova & Thalhauser, 2011) is unique in each person, making planning for adapting changes difficult for families. Periodic disruptions in family routines and rituals as well as changes in the perceived demands/capabilities ratio occur as existing stressors unfold and as new stressors emerge (Harrist, Henry, Liu, & Morris, in press). Thus, managing cycles of greater and lesser caregiving demands often become a natural part of on-going family life, requiring changes in family demands within fairly short time frames.

1.1.1.2 Protection and Vulnerabilities

A premise of the FRM is that families have capabilities (or strengths) that can serve as the foundation for protection against the potential negative outcomes of significant risk (Patterson, 2002; Walsh, 2012a). Family protection encompasses both the existing and new strengths of families that help them successfully navigate risk in ways that individual family members, family subsystems, overall family systems, and interfaces with the family-proximal (or close) ecosystem function adequately (Henry et al., 2015). Internal family strengths and a positive interface with proximal ecosystems, such as support through family and friends as well as the medical and social services communities, can protect against caregiving risks, increasing the potential for family resilience (Martin, Distelberg, & Elahad, 2015). In turn, families and their members often redefine (or reframe) difficult caregiving situations to make them more manageable such that a "new normal" emerges, potentially yielding competent functioning in both the short- and long-term.

Protection involves both promotive and protective processes. Promotive processes support competence when significant risk is not present while protective processes facilitate resilience or competence when significant risk is present (Masten & Monn, 2015). Before significant caregiving risk, a positive outlook is promotive, helping families fulfill their functions with competence whereas a positive outlook during caregiving is protection as it is employed to cope with changes in the needs of a care recipient, reduce the tension between family members, foster quality communication, and increase the potential for positive family adaptation.

Because caregiving stressors rarely occur as the only source of stress in a family system, other vulnerabilities often co-occur, yielding a pile-up of stressors (Patterson, 2012). Vulnerabilities are other vertical or horizontal stressors beyond the focal stressor that heighten the risk for negative outcomes (Henry et al., 2015). A family member of an individual in need of an in-depth dementia evaluation may have significant difficulty addressing this need due to other family or work demands. A spouse may delay or avoid the evaluation, driven by loyalty to protect the spouse from the reality of bad news or fear that a diagnosis might result in lifestyle changes (e.g., moving out of the family home or giving up independence). Pre-existing vulnerabilities from earlier life stages and roles may come into greater focus as family members seek to work together to address caregiving needs. For example, childlessness, adult child challenges (e.g., job stress, transitions), or unresolved parent-child issues heighten family risk. Likewise, an adult child may find putting aside on-going relationship strain is necessary to implementing medical power of attorney for a parent to assure adequate care.

Family protection and vulnerability depends, in part, upon on-going interaction patterns in caregiver-care recipient subsystems, other family subsystems, overall family systems, and family–proximal ecosystem interfaces. Current interaction patterns may no longer work as new caregiving challenges arise. Some family system qualities such as flexibility, or adapting expectations and behavior to correspond to current realities, tend to offer protection as care system needs increase (Martin et al., 2017). Family issues such as concurrent illnesses of multiple family members increase vulnerability, making caregiving more complex. Interestingly, some aspects of protection and vulnerability are the negative and positive poles of the same quality (Rutter, 1987). For example, caregiver self-efficacy, or perceived ability to organize and execute caregiving, protects against stress and burden when high and increases vulnerability when low (Johnson, Wolfteich, & Harrell, 2014). The geographic proximity of caregivers and care recipients also may influence protection or vulnerabilities. Closer proximity of caregivers to care recipients may increase assistance with both activities of daily living (ADLs) and instrumental activities of daily living (IADLs) (Bevan & Sparks, 2011) whereas long distance caregivers may be more likely to assist only with IADLs, such as financial management (Koerin & Harrigan, 2003). Long distance family caregivers are more likely than their geographically closer counterparts to miss age-associated changes that show signs of needing care or have difficulty locating services due to a lack of familiarity with the area, while proximal caregivers may resent long distance caregivers who are viewed as not doing enough (Bevan & Sparks, 2011; Koerin & Harrigan, 2003). Assessing changing caregiving needs for family members with progressive cognitive disorders can be challenging (Bailey & Gordon, 2016). Yet, effective family communication, organization, and coherence, individual independence and self-esteem, and social support hold potential to protect and when mobilized to navigate caregiving stress (McCubbin & Patterson, 1983). Resilience-oriented interventions for caregiving families can be designed to reduce family vulnerables by increasing their capacity "in dealing with crises, navigating disruptive transitions, weathering persistent stresses, and meeting future challenges" (Walsh, 2012b, p. 156).

1.1.1.3 Adaptation

Adaptation describes how well family systems fulfill their fundamental functions during and after family caregiving and takes into account the meaning that arises to family members about the risk, protection, and vulnerabilities (Henry et al., 2015; McCubbin & Patterson, 1983; Patterson, 2002). Proximal care systems (e.g., medical and social service services) tend to emphasize care recipients and, to some degree, caregivers and available access to medical or social services. Yet, competent caregiving occurs as care recipients interface with and between other family members, family subsystems, overall family system, and proximal ecosystems of care services throughout the many, often frequent changes associated with the ebb and flow of caregiving needs and stressors over time (Henry et al., 2015; Patterson, 2002; Walsh, 2012b).

Adaptation to caregiving is an on-going process that involves effectively navigating multiple caregiving stressors at multiple system levels in both the short- and long-term. Both short- and long-term adaptation occur on a continuum with the anchors of bonadaptation and maladaptation (McCubbin & Patterson, 1983). Bonadaptation (or positive adaptation) to caregiving stressors is evident as families function competently (or adequate), consistent with capabilities in each part of the system. Long-term bonadaptation can involve a "steeling effect" (Rutter, 2013, p. 477) where a family becomes less vulnerable to potential negative outcomes of future caregiving stressors due to "inoculation" of, or adaptation to current stressors. Bonadaptation can involve growth from positively navigating caregiving stressors, often with specific families growing (or building promotive capacity) in some areas of functioning while functioning adequately in other areas and still yield competence (McCubbin & Patterson, 1983; Walsh, 2012a). Yet, bonadaptation only requires competence, not necessarily growth since resilience, by definition involves competence despite risk (Wright et al., 2013). Maladaptation (or negative family adaptation) occurs as one or more parts of a family system fail to recalibrate to changes such that adequate functioning emerges, often contributing to a pile-up of stressors including new and existing vulnerabilities or an additional crisis (McCubbin & Patterson, 1983; Patterson, 2002). To assess whether adequate functioning is present across multiple family system levels requires consideration of how competence may be manifested in individual family members, family subsystems, overall family systems, and the family-proximal ecosystem (or care system) interface.

Adequately addressing the needs of care recipients, caregivers, and other family members is critical to family adaptation to aspects of family caregiving. Adaptation involves each family member showing competence in developmental tasks consistent with their capabilities despite challenges. For example, consider a family member with dementia for whom adaptation includes adequate functioning relative to the neurobiological, cognitive, psychosocial, and contextual capabilities associated with the current stage of dementia (see Table 1.1). The degenerative nature of dementia yields decline over time. Thus, bonadaptation of a person with dementia may involve comfort and safety, preserving the sense of personhood and dignity, competence in key areas of life consistent with their current capabilities and circumstances (including culture), and renegotiating relationships to accept dependence on others, navigating interfaces with proximal ecosystems, and coming to terms with mortality in the self and others (McCormick, Kuo, & Masten, 2011; Walsh, 2012b).

Family subsystems are an integral part of family adaptation. In family caregiving, adaptation involves adequately meeting current caregiving demands, coordinating with other caregivers such as informal and formal medical and service providers, and managing each members' (e.g., biological, cultural, contextual) and the family systems' (e.g., young adults leaving home) developmentally appropriate tasks in key domains (McCormick et al., 2011; McGoldrick & Shibusawa, 2012). Consider how a couple subsystem changes when a spouse assumes caregiving for a spouse with dementia. Caregiving demands and the declining abilities of the spouse with dementia can begin with adding caregiving responsibilities and taking on roles formerly performed by the spouse. Over time, the ambiguous loss of former patterns of intimacy result in ambiguous loss where the caregiving spouse sees their spouse as physically present, yet psychologically absent (Boss, 1993). In turn, coping may involve redefining the relationship as more as a caregiver and less as a spouse (Boss, 1993).

Other family subsystems also may change. An adult child or grandchild may assume responsibility for coordinating the interface between a parent who is a care recipient and proximal caregivers which may, in turn, not only change parent-adult child and couple subsystems or other subsystems (e.g., sibling relations among adult children). As specific health stressors arise, caregivers may focus on managing the immediate needs of the care recipient rather than their own needs or those of other family members. Family systems may experience significant risk if one person assumes the majority of caregiving responsibilities without rebalancing other key roles in the family or workplace. In turn, overall family systems often require recalibration to make changes in who does what in families. Without such change, over time, family vulnerabilities may increase as the caregiver becomes less competent in fulfilling family functions including caregiving or develop health symptoms. Subsystems may experience change to increase the coordination across to mobilize the collective family system resources for protection when risk is present (Walsh, 2012b).

At the overall family system level, families fulfill functions for society and their members including membership and family formation, economic support, nurturance and socialization, and protection of vulnerable members (Patterson, 2002). This occurs through family adaptive systems (described in a later section) that develop and regulate family emotions, roles and rules, worldviews and identities, regulate the capacity to meet basic needs, and the ability to adapt to changing needs within the family system (Harrist et al., in press; Henry et al., 2015). Yet, competent overall family system functioning (or positive outcomes) differs over time as the intensity of care challenges varies over time. For example, greater family cohesiveness facilitates the progression through specific stressors, while facilitating greater autonomy during stable phases (Walsh, 2012b). Further, overall family system adaptation is intertwined with competent functioning in family subsystems, individuals, and the interface of families with proximal ecosystem resources involved in caregiving.

1.1.1.4 Family Situational Meanings

Family situational meanings are overall family shared appraisals of specific stressors that emerge through interaction. These meanings develop in the contexts of family worldviews and identity. Significant risk, protection, vulnerabilities, and adaptation occur in concert with family situational meanings. Individual family members do not always agree upon situational meanings, yet collective family system meanings emerge when families share their experiences with each other and form a collective meaning (Patterson & Garwick, 1994). Family caregiving experiences offer the potential for reappraisals of life priorities and new insights (Walsh, 2012b). Resilience in family caregiving requires redefining (or reframing) caregiving challenges in meaningful and manageable ways (Boss, 1993, 2010). Thus, families can move from a deficit-focused view of caregiving toward goals such as growth through adversity, effective coping, and problem solving (Patterson, 2002).

Alzheimer's disease and other forms of dementia present a situation where shared family beliefs inhibit resilience. The ambivalence and ambiguity accompanying the disease processes as well as the lack of consensus between disciplines

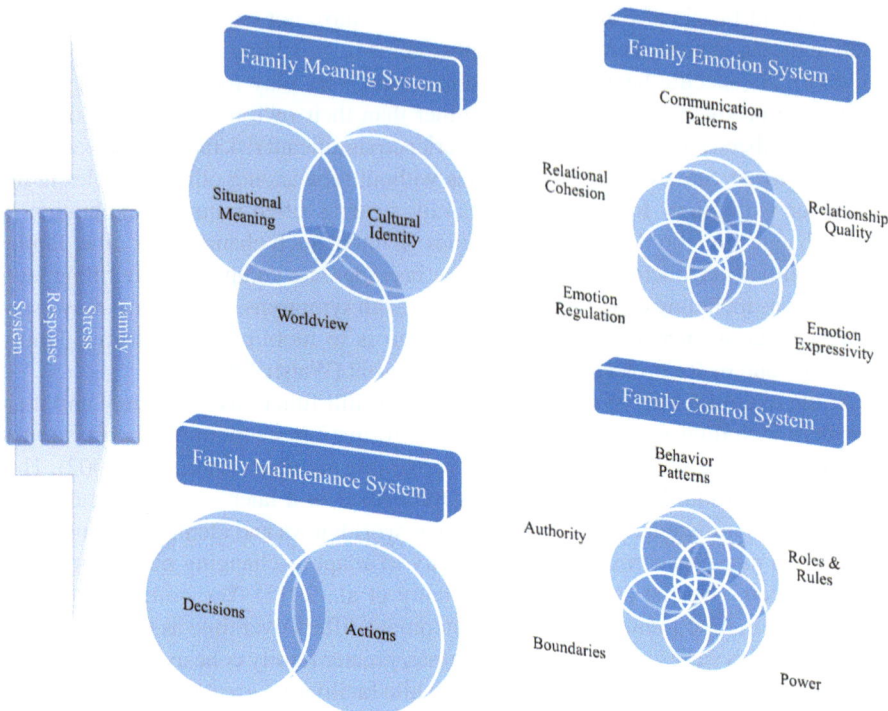

Fig. 1.3 Family adaptive systems

regarding stages of progression make developing shared family meaning difficult (Boss, 2010; Sarazin, Horne, & Dubois, 2007). Short-and long-term adaptation are likely to be enhanced through redefining such challenges in ways that offer hope, optimism, and meaning that increase manageability (Hellman, Worley, & Munoz, this volume; Walsh, 2012a, 2012b). Caregiving risks increase the likelihood of maladaptation, at least in the short-term. Yet, the current or new capabilities of families can afford protection that increase the potential of competent functioning despite caregiving risks. On-going risks, developmental changes in families, or a pile-up of stressors can occur that compound the risk. In addition, it is critical to recognize the subjective nature of risk, protection, vulnerability, and adaptation. Overall, the situational meanings family members construct about caregiver risks, protection, vulnerability, and adaptation are critical to understanding how families navigate caregiving experiences.

A tenant of the FRM is that applying the core resilience concepts described above to family caregiving requires consideration of how these occur in concert with complex family adaptive systems (see Fig. 1.3) and ecosystems. In this section, we define family adaptive systems and discuss the maintenance, meaning, emotion, control, and stress response systems.

1.1.2 Family Adaptive Systems

Family protection, vulnerability, and adaptation occur in concert with family adaptive systems (Harrist et al., in press; Henry et al., 2015). Parallel to human adaptive systems including health and stress, information processing and problem solving, and attachment that promote individual resilience (Wright et al., 2013), *family adaptive systems* (FAS) emerge within family systems (Henry et al., 2015). Complex FAS help families fulfill their functions for family and society (Henry et al. 2015; Patterson, 2002). FAS characterize on-going family relationship patterns around family functions, yielding behavioral patterns with expectations and acceptable behavioral variations. FAS may offer protection or heighten vulnerability as well as representing domains of short- and long-term adaptation to significant risk (Henry et al., 2015). FAS work in tandem with each other to promote competency in family functioning. FAS vary from family to family in terms of ability to foster competence before, during, and after caregiving. Specific indicators of adaptation within the FAS range from positive (bonadaptation) to negative (maladaptation) and are evident at each family system level (Henry et al., 2015).

In this section, we discuss selected FAS involved in resilience for families engaged in caregiving (see Table 1.2). Collectively, family adaptive systems emerge around family functions that are important to individual family members and society including, but not necessarily limited to, maintenance, emotion, control, meaning, and managing stress that disrupt ongoing interaction patterns. Through family interactions, FAS emerge to regulate family dynamics as families navigate the challenges of day-to-day interactions, including family caregiving, along with daily hassles, individual and family developmental changes and unpredictable stress (Henry et al., 2015). In Fig. 1.3, the family maintenance, meaning, and emotion systems are encompassing multiple dimensions, while the stress response system is an underlying system that balances stability and change in each of the other FAS.

1.1.2.1 Family Maintenance Systems

Family maintenance systems are family interaction patterns that arise to meet and maintain basic needs for food, clothing, shelter, health, and related issues, such as financial management. In family caregiving, the individual caregivers assist with ADLs and IADLs, gain medical and financial assistance, deal with legal issues such as power of attorney or estates, and provide emotional support. While one caregiver focuses on assisting the care recipient, other family members may provide assistance to both the caregiver(s) and care recipient such as cooking meals a few times a week or grocery shopping. For couples engaging in mutual caregiving, support in the extended family system is particularly important. Authors in this volume (Hermann & Struckmeyer, this volume; Jayadas & Kang, this volume; Schroeder & Osteen, this volume) discuss aspects of protection and vulnerability relating to nutrition, ergonomics, and finances.

Table 1.2 Application of Family Adaptive Systems at multiple levels to spousal caregiving

		Emotion system	Control system	Meaning system	Maintenance system	Stress response
Care recipient	Bonadaptation	Self-soothing and seeking emotional support	Balancing needs for control with needs for assistance	Constructing a meaning that separates self from the condition	Independent functioning and/or accepting care consistent with medical, food, and shelter needs	Adjusts individual coping to balance stability and adaptability needs
	Maladaptation	Over reliance on others to organize emotions; emotional isolation	Over or under functioning in life decisions	Seeing self as burden or as deficient as a person	Inadequate ability or gain needed medical, food, and shelter needs	Hyperarousal of the SNS and HPA-axis[a]; inability to maintain stability or to adapt
Caregiver	Bonadaptation	Self-soothing and seeking emotional support	Self-regulating and influencing decision making process	Integrating caregiving roles into identity	Ability for and access to self-care; sufficient resources for medical, food, and shelter needs	Adjusts individual coping to balance stability and adaptability needs
	Maladaptation	Over reliance on others to organize emotions; emotional isolation	Holding onto previous patterns of decision making and power	Inadequately modifying identity integrating past and present; seeing declines as one's inadequacy as a caregiver	Restricted accessibility; time; or skills to assure well-being for both self and care recipient	Hyperarousal of the SNS and HPA-axis; inability to maintain stability or to adapt

		Emotion system	Control system	Meaning system	Maintenance system	Stress response
Couple	*Bonadaptation*	Ability to express emotional needs during the progression of illness to spouse	Roles, rules and boundaries are able to shift appropriately between partners	Beliefs are realistic about the progression of the disease. Caregiving viewed as an extension of the relationship	Relationship continues to be a priority and interactions continue the care giver/recipient relationship to the degree possible	Couple interactions provide a sense of stability and incorporate needed adjustments as the disease progresses
	Maladaptation	Inability to express disappointment; seeing each other more negatively than positively	Rigid or diffused roles unable to adapt to the progression of the diagnosis	Viewing spouse as object; seeing caregiving is a futile effort	Medical, food, or shelter needs neglected; couple interactions primarily on giving/receiving care when not medically necessary	Couple interactions increase stress levels that prolong the activation of SNS and HPA
Overall family system	*Bonadaptation*	Emotional needs shared across the generations; caring and connection rituals modified as needed	Appropriate boundaries between sub-systems	Sense of generativity and reciprocity	Mobilizing resources across sub-systems to meet financial, food, and shelter needs	Maintaining a balance between stability while adapting to changes during progression of condition
	Maladaptation	Emotional over-load or limited emotional expression between spouses or generations; putting rituals on indefinite hold	Disengaged or enmeshed relationships between sub systems	Learned hopelessness	Difficulty providing adequate financial, housing, and food needs across the generations	Rigid coping that restricts adaption or stability; over accommodation to condition

(continued)

Table 1.2 (continued)

		Emotion system	Control system	Meaning system	Maintenance system	Stress response
Family-proximal ecosystem (F-PEI) interface	Bonadaptation	F-PEI provides emotional support	Well-functioning F-PEI in caregiving decisions	Family viewed as important part of the F-PEI	F-PEI provides support for housing, food, and financial needs	Community members model appropriate stress regulation
	Maladaptation	Limited family emotional support in F-PEI	Rigid or diffused boundaries in the F-PEI e	Family disconnected from and unfamiliar with proximal resources	F-PEI does not provide adequate housing, food, and financial needs are met	Poor neighborhood quality that promotes increased biological stress arousal

[a]The sympathetic nervous system (SNS) stimulates the fight or flight response, while the hypothalamic-pituitary-adrenal axis (HPA-axis) is the body's central stress response system that regulates the endocrine system release of stress hormones (e.g., cortisol)

1.1.2.2 Family Meaning Systems

Family meaning systems emerge through sharing time, space, and communication with three inter-related components: *family worldview, family identity, and meaning making* (Patterson & Garwick, 1994). The *family worldview* describes family members' shared assumptions about and interpretations of their environment, and beliefs about their purpose and place in life (Patterson & Garwick, 1994). Aspects of ethnicity and culture integrate into the meaning systems of specific families (McCubbin & McCubbin, 2013). Family worldviews likely to afford protection to caregiving families include: (a) a *shared purpose* (e.g., perceived needs of the care recipient), (b) a *collective approach* (e.g., common goals combined with *shared control* or trust with healthcare providers), (c) *frameability* (e.g., integrating optimism and hope with reality), (d) *relativism* (e.g., living flexibly in the present), and (e) *spirituality* (e.g., seeing challenges in relation to a higher power or nature) (Patterson, 1988; Walsh, 2012a). Spirituality, for example, holds strong potential for assisting families in creating redefining caregiving in ways to be more manageable (Martin et al., 2015).

Family identity describes shared themes that serve as the basis for organizing family life to reduce ambiguity and foster boundaries regarding who participates and how they participate in families (Patterson & Garwick, 1994). Themes emerge in concert with family worldviews and culture, representing shared beliefs and expectations about aspects of family life such as parenting, couple relationships, education, occupation, religious views, status, or cultural identity. Family legacies of values, social identity, or family rituals involve themes in families that continue from prior generations (Boszormenyi-Nagy & Sparks, 1973; Reiss, 1981; Walsh, 2012a). Families often have themes about who should provide care and in what ways (e.g., the oldest daughter will be the primary caregiver) and engage in caregiving long before developing a collective identity including caregiving (Qualls & Williams, 2013). Together, family worldviews and identities comprise the meaning system that interacts with other FAS as families appraise and make meaning of specific caregiving challenges.

1.1.2.3 Family Control Systems

Family control systems describe complex patterns of authority (rules, roles and power), organization, and behavior (day-to-day interactions, expectations (stated or unstated) for how things "should" be in the family system, often boundaries) in family systems. These patterns arise through interaction involving rules or influenced by family heritage, culture, religious, or other norms. Family routines and rituals arise that guide daily interactions and bring families together to recognize traditions and special occasions (Harrist et al., in press; McCubbin & McCubbin, 1991). Caregiving demands often disrupt long-standing patterns of interaction governing control due to new family responsibilities associated with caregiving. When one spouse cares for the other spouse, a spouse who always had decision-making authority over finances may now need assistance, requiring a transfer of this authority to the other spouse or an adult child (see Table 1.1, Qualls & Williams, 2013). The complexity of orchestrating control increases as multiple caregivers provide care for the same care recipient.

> **Breakout Box 1.1 Focus on Practice**
> As a caregiver for my elderly mother, who died at 97, and now my husband, who has Alzheimer's disease and dementia, I can attest to the stressors faced by caregivers, particularly those of immigrant background. My mother, born in South America, came to live with me in the United States when my only child was born. She helped me take care of my daughter, which greatly ameliorated the stressors I faced as a working mom. As my mother grew older, she lived an independent life; however, the activities she could do without my help were limited by her low English language proficiency. I was my mother's only child. My husband, who was born in Europe, has no close relatives either. Our adult daughter lives in a different city. I care for my husband at home and plan to continue doing so for as long as I am able. In Latino cultures, we take care of our loved ones at home instead of institutionalizing them. We feel it is our moral obligation and an honor to take care of those who have been there for us. Taking care of our elders at home gives us satisfaction and a sense of accomplishment. At the same time, caring for younger or elderly family members without a strong support system is challenging. The absence of a network of family members with whom to share caregiving duties for my mother and my husband, the language barriers faced by my mother, and my husband's physical and social isolation at home are the main stressors I have experienced as a caregiver. Because I still work, my husband was spending significant amounts of time alone at home. Out of concern for his safety, I invited a friend who does odd jobs to live with us. I would like to find an adult day center that provides social activities for people with Alzheimer's dementia. My religious faith and values, acceptance of my husband's condition, as well as focusing on the joy my husband still derives from life's little things and moments have been a source of resilience as a caregiver.
> —*Ms. Irma Chajecki, Community Volunteer.*

Families use three primary control strategies for caregiving (Davis, 1997). *Substitutive caregiving* occurs as families identify one caregiver believed to be most able to provide care and other family members fill in only as needed. *Complementary caregiving* involves a primary caregiver accompanied by other family members providing supportive practical assistance (e.g., running errands, personal care, managing finances, or completing household chores). *Conjoint caregiving* involves multiple family members that partner in ongoing care (Davis, 1997). Family control systems that allow for flexibility in roles, rules, power, organization, or approaches to caregiving afford protection to caregiving families (Henry et al., 2015;

Martin et al., 2015). In contrast, rigidity in these qualities may increase the vulnerability to negative outcomes.

1.1.2.4 Family Emotion Systems

Family emotion systems regulate the emotional climate or interaction patterns encompassing expressivity, emotion regulation, communication patterns, relationship quality, and connectedness. Family emotion systems, often evident through family communication patterns, range from cooperative to competitive (Speice, Shields, & Blieszner, 1998). Families with cooperative emotion systems afford protection through qualities such as healthy family communication patterns (clarity, open emotional sharing, collaborative problem solving), balancing connectedness and autonomy, family member accord, time together, family coherence and unity, mutual recreational interests, social support beyond the family, and efforts to build family emotional capabilities (Black & Lobo, 2008; McCubbin & Patterson, 1983; Walsh, 2012a). A cooperative emotion system allows family members to work effectively to address challenges. In contrast, a competitive emotion system may enhance vulnerabilities through interactions characterized by criticism, defensiveness, hostility, or trying to "one-up" each other, creating difficulties in the regulation of anger or sadness that are common in caregiving families.

1.1.2.5 Family Stress Response Systems

The family stress response system (FSRS) regulates the other FAS such as the maintenance, identity, emotion, and control systems when on-going family dynamics are disrupted by stress to restore stability or establish modified interaction patterns (see Fig. 1.3). The FSRS is analogous to the biological stress systems which activate a complex series of hormonal responses to stress through which chronic stress adapt through increased release of hormones, heightening the risk for negative adaptation with potential to yield immune deficiencies, damage to the hippocampus, cognitive impairment, or adjustment problems (Ha & Granger, 2016). Effectively addressing biological stress fosters positive adaptation or a new steady state promoting health and resilience. In families, the response system regulates deviations from on-going interaction patterns in the FAS, increasing or attenuating risk.

As a care recipient needs assistance, the disruption in the balance in family interaction occurs, at least temporarily. Yet, prolonged caregiving can result in chronic stress that can be temporary and addressed through modifications in one or more FAS to restore balance and adaptation. Alternatively, chronic stress can result in a longer disruption in balance in each family adaptive system whereby family members perceive an on-going state of family demands outweighing family capabilities. In families with heightened vulnerability before assuming caregiving, the transition into caregiving activates the FSRS in ways that compromise the on-going interaction patterns that regulate the maintenance, identity, emotion, and control systems just as the biological stress systems respond to physiological stress. For example, when families view caregiving activities simply as part of an on-going family theme (e.g., "we take care of each other") without recognizing the added responsibilities may find it difficult to achieve a sense of balance (or a "new normal") in the maintenance, meaning, or control systems. In turn, these changes stress the family emotion system though changes such as decreased emotion regulation in relationships between family members. As families become aware of caregiving stressors, the other FAS employ the FSRS to either restore stability in or establish a new steady state by modifying ongoing family interaction patterns. Successfully navigating pressure on the FAS plays a critical role in the abilities of families to adapt to significant risks of caregiving.

1.1.3 Distal and Proximal Ecosystem Fit

Distal ecosystems, or the biological, physical, and social environments of families, are critical to understanding caregiving as they regulate the resources and support available to families at multiple levels of social systems. Not only do individuals and families adapt to caregiving, aspects of the environment can adapt to either reduce risk or limit the negative consequences of risk. The family-home health care system, for example, might modify the scheduling of visits to honor religious or cultural traditions that differ from the broader culture. The goodness of fit between families and proximal ecosystems is central to assuring the well-being of care recipients and their families during an often-challenging journey. Distal ecosystems such as healthcare and social systems regulate polices and funding that are critical for assuring the availability of care services in local communities (see Roberts, this volume) relevant to challenges such as increased numbers of long distance caregivers associated with global market expansion, demographic trends (baby boomers, longevity, declining birth rates), and work obligations (Cagle & Munn, 2012).

1.2 Implications

In this chapter, we build on earlier scholarship conceptualizing caregiving as both a family system (Qualls & Williams, 2013) and a family resilience issue (Walsh, 2012b), showing the utility of the FRM as a conceptual tool for understanding how family resilience occurs in caregiving families. Family caregiving risk is two-fold since caregiving status involves risk and caregiving involves specific stressors, often involving transitions, leaving families feeling an imbalance between their capabilities (protection) and demands (risks and vulnerabilities). Yet, through processes such as mobilizing existing strengths and accessing new resources as well as redefining situations, families have the potential to show competent functioning despite caregiving risk. Communities with strong healthcare and social service capabilities focusing on supporting families caring for adult family members imply policies and funding that take family needs into account).

This chapter extends existing scholarship by bridging caregiving and family resilience scholarship across multiple family system levels: individual family members (including, but not limited to, caregivers and care recipients), subsystems, overall family systems, and the interface between families and proximal ecosystems. Because the nature of caregiving often requires interfaces with proximal ecosystems (e.g., healthcare) and the disproportionate focus on individual over family caregiving, we modified the FRM to specifically locate the multiple system levels at the center of the core family resilience concepts. Thus, policy-makers, program directors, family members, and others may refer to this visual reminder of the multiple system levels involved in family caregiving.

1.2.1 Implications: A Case Study

To illustrate how aspects of the FRM apply to working directly with specific families, we offer a case study describing the involvement of FAS in family caregiving and resilience. At the heart of caregiving is the specific condition(s) of the care recipient. Caregiving may involve developmental progressions in family members (e.g., transitioning young adults with intellectual and developmental disabilities into community living arrangements), or an overall trajectory of decline. Declines can occur in varying patterns over time (e.g., linear or curvilinear), vary between individuals, and vary in progression and intensity. The following family case study involves dementia diagnosis for one member (see Table 1.1).

Martina Alvarez (a 70-year-old woman) was recently diagnosed with dementia. Her 75-year-old husband, José has been struggling with diabetes and high blood pressure for several years. Before starting a family, Martina and José immigrated to the United States from Mexico for José to work with a company based in Tulsa, Oklahoma, and eventually became United States citizens. Beyond José and Martina, family members include three adult children: José Jr. (married to Emily, a Caucasian woman, and three adolescent children), Maria (married to Paul, a third generation Mexican American man, and five children ranging in age from 5 to 17), and Camila (divorced, working, no children, and struggles with alcoholism) (see Fig. 1.4 for a brief genogram). The couple, their adult children, and grandchildren all live in Tulsa. Martina and José's parents passed away a few years ago in Mexico where their extended families remain. The couple has long-term close friendships in their church (family-ecosystem fit). José and Martina have a long tradition of marital satisfaction, having shared the transition to a new country, raised three children, and developed relationships with other immigrant families and the broader community.

Due to their age and Martina's recent Alzheimer's diagnosis, José had the cultural expectation (meaning system) that they would move in with José Jr. and his family. José Jr.'s wife already feels overwhelmed with her responsibilities taking care of her husband and their three teenagers, as well as her part-time job to support

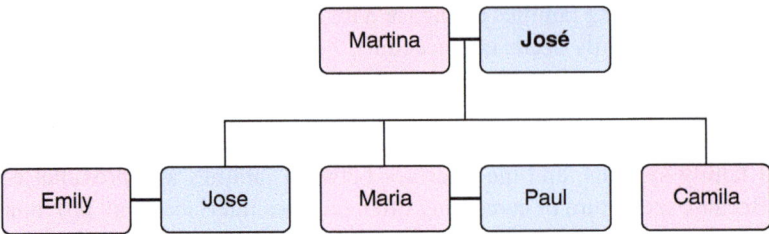

Fig. 1.4 Genogram of Alvarez family

the family's financial demands (maintenance system). Upon learning that they could not live with José Jr., Martina expressed a strong desire to continue living in their own home (control system) and have her children provide support to José in providing care (control system). Maria and Paul insisted they move into their home on a temporary basis. José arranged for Martina's niece Mayda to fly in from Mexico to care for Martina (meaning and control systems). Mayda left her job to care for her beloved aunt and to fulfill traditions of extended kin ties to care for Martina (maintenance and meaning systems). Mayda took over doing the shopping, cooking, laundry, and finances, while Martina continued to do some housekeeping (maintenance system). José continued his role as family provider and decision maker. The children and their families regularly came to the home to assure family traditions continued and that José and Martina had the support they needed (emotion system).

Over time, Martina's condition progressed and José began to help Mayda in assisting Martina in meeting her ADLs (maintenance system). Because of the stress of decline of his wife, the responsibility he felt, and the demands of caregiving, José's health declined to the point where José Jr. assumed durable power of attorney for both of his parents. The Alvarez family (the couple and their adult children and spouses) decided to have Camila move in with José and Martina (control system). Camila was able to provide caregiving support to Martina and José as well as emotional support as they worried about disease progression (emotion system). Other family members provided care to allow Camila time away from caregiving two afternoons a week. This shows the family stress response system allowing for adaptation in the family maintenance system to allow for changes in the emotion, control, and meaning systems while adhering to the family value of *familiso*, or maintaining connectedness to and responsibility in the family system, while supporting the long-term marital commitment of Jose and Martina (meaning system). This allowed Martina and José to remain in their home with family solidarity supporting their needs (family stress response system).

The Alvarez family continues to face challenges that trigger the FSRS as caregiving risks increase due to disease progression and a pile-up of stressors. In turn, the family redefines the situation with each change to make shifts that accommodate the new, often unexpected and arduous process of modifying caregiving approaches, often involving greater interfaces with the proximal-ecosystem (healthcare and social services). Cultural strengths such as *familiso* and *respecto* hold potential for greater openness in the couple system to allow multiple generations of their family to provide support in ways that recognize the tradition of parental authority, responsibility, and connectedness among family members (meaning system). Such qualities can be particularly beneficial when the FSRS allows for flexibility in meeting the healthcare needs of the older generation (maintenance system) while modifying existing traditions in ways that meet the current demands and honor the parents (meaning and emotion systems).

1.2.2 Implications for Policy and Practice

In this chapter, we applied the Family Resilience Model (Henry et al., 2015) to caregiving to illustrate how individual family members (care recipients, caregivers, and other family members), family subsystems (spouses or partners, parent-adult child relationships, siblings, grandparent-grandchild), overall family systems, and family-proximal ecosystems interface in resilient family caregiving. Family caregiving may be most effective when risk, protection and vulnerabilities, and situational meanings using a view of as interfacing with FAS and distal ecosystems, and when competent functioning or adaptation occurs at each system level. In this volume, authors provide examples and future directions for pursuing aspects of family resilience and caregiving relating to specific aspects of the FRM. Notably, caregiving of adult family members with cognitive, physical, or psychological challenges comprise this volume. Despite our examples' focus on older adults, our ideas apply to caregiving for across the life cycle including young adults and children with intellectual or developmental disabilities.

Policymakers and practitioners are encouraged to follow these principles from family resilience, including the application of the FRM to caregiving (see Henry et al., 2015; Qualls & Williams, 2013; Walsh, 2012b).

1. *Family system dynamics are critical to the well-being of care recipients.* Thus, policies are critical that recognize caregiving as part of family system dynamics. Practitioners can start by identifying the family system members (spouses, partners, children, stepchildren, grandchildren, stepgrandchildren, extended family, and affiliated kin).
2. *Families appraise and develop situational meaning about caregiving risk, protection, vulnerability, and adaptation.* The process of adapting to change often involves family members creating modified collective definitions of the situation that arise through interaction, informed by family worldviews (e.g., culture, religion) and family identity as well as specific stressors.
3. *At any point in the caregiving process, families have both strengths that hold potential to afford protection and other vulnerabilities embedded in on-going family adaptive systems.* Family adaptive systems arise as complex sets of interaction patterns focused on functional areas in families including emotion, control, meaning, maintenance, and stress response. Practitioners often work with families to identify and mobilize family strengths to facilitate caregiving in ways that also foster family system well-being.

4. *Effective family caregiving involves positive family-ecosystem fit.* Proximal ecosystems that provide services that tailored to interface well with specific families and occur within distal ecosystems relevant to both families (e.g., culture) and society (e.g., policy, or social trends).

Questions for Thought and Discussion

1. Using the Family Resilience Model for caregiving, compare and contrast how the family caregiving can be described and assessed at each of the following family system levels: individual family members, subsystems, the overall family system, and the family-proximal ecosystem fit.
2. Share an example of horizontal and vertical stressors and potential subsequent "pile up" of stressors that might occur at multiple levels of family systems engaged in caregiving.
3. Describe examples of how family adaptive systems may interact to foster family resilience in family caregiving.
4. Give examples promoting the family resilience trajectory toward bonadaptation as well as advancing toward maladaptation.
5. Consider the family caregiving scenario of a couple where one member has dementia characterized by a steady and unremitting deterioration of cognitive, emotional, relational, and physical functioning. Using Table 1.1, discuss and give examples of how protective processes and vulnerabilities may evolve and change as the condition progresses.
6. As a medical or social service provider, how might you interface with caregiving families to offer relevant and beneficial assistance in their journey toward resilience?

References

Alzheimer's Association. (2016). *Stages of Alzheimer's*. Retrieved from http://www.alz.org/alzheimers_disease_stages_of_alzheimers.asp

Alzheimer's Society. (2016). *The progression of Alzheimer's disease and other dementias*. Retrieved from https://www.alzheimers.org.uk/site/scripts/documents_info.php?documentID=133

Bailey, W. A., & Gordon, S. R. (2016). Family caregiving amidst age-associated cognitive changes: Implications for practice and future generations. *Family Relations, 65*, 225–238. doi:10.1111/fare.12176

Bevan, J. L., & Sparks, L. (2011). Communication in the context of long-distance family caregiving: An integrated review and practical applications. *Patient Education and Counseling, 85*, 26–30. doi:10.1016/j.pec.2010.08.003

Black, K., & Lobo, M. (2008). A conceptual review of family resilience factors. *Journal of Family Nursing, 14*, 33–55. doi:10.1177/1074840707312237

Boss, P. (1993). The reconstruction of family life with Alzheimer's disease: Generating theory to lower family risk from ambiguous loss. In P. Boss, W. J. Dougherty, R. LaRossa, W. R. Schumm, & S. K. Steinmetz (Eds.), *Family theories and methods* (pp. 163–166). New York, NY: Plenum.

Boss, P. (2010). The trauma and complicated grief of ambiguous loss. *Pastoral Psychology, 59*, 137–145. doi:10.1007/s11089-009-0264-0

Boszormenyi-Nagy, I., & Sparks, G. (1973). *Invisible loyalties.* New York, NY: Harper & Rowe.
Cagle, J. G., & Munn, J. C. (2012). Long-distance caregiving: A systematic review of the literature. *Journal of Gerontological Social Work, 55,* 682–707. doi:10.1080/01634372.2012.703763
Cornille, T. A., & Boroto, D. R. (1992). The Family Distress Model: A conceptual and clinical application of Reiss' strong bonds finding. *Contemporary Family Therapy, 14,* 181–198. doi:10.1007/bf00901503
Davis, L. L. (1997). Family conflicts around dementia home-care. *Families, Systems, & Health, 15,* 85–98. doi:10.1037/h0089810
Ha, T., & Granger, D. A. (2016). Family relations, stress, and vulnerability: Biobehavioral implications for prevention and practice. *Family Relations, 65,* 9–23. doi:10.1111/fare.12173
Haley, W. E. (2003). The costs of family caregiving: Implications for geriatric oncology. *Critical Reviews in Oncology and Hematology, 48,* 151–158. doi:10.1016/j.critrevonc.2003.04.005
Harrist, A. W., Henry, C. S., Liu, C., & Morris, A. S. (forthcoming). Family resilience: The power of rituals and routines in family adaptive systems. In B. H. Fiese (Ed.), The APA handbook of contemporary family psychology: Foundations, methods, and changing forms, Volume 1. Washington, DC: American Psychological Association Press.
Hellman, C., Worley, J. A., & Munoz, R. T. (this volume). Caregiver well-being: Hope as a coping resource.
Henry, C. S., Morris, A. S., & Harrist, A. W. (2015). Family resilience: Moving into the third wave. *Family Relations, 64,* 22–43. doi:10.1111/fare.12106
Hermann, J., & Struckmeyer, K. M. (this volume). Older adult caregivers: Older adult nutrition, meals, and food safety.
Jayadas, A., & Kang, M. (this volume). Improving ergonomics for the safety, comfort and health of caregivers.
Johnson, E. L., Wolfteich, P. M., & Harrell, T. H. (2014). Differences in caregiver self-efficacy and satisfaction related to sexual abuse of offspring. *Journal of Child Sexual Abuse, 23,* 504–518. doi:10.1080/10538712.2014.919370
Johnston, J. H., Bailey, W. A., & Wilson, G. (2014). Mechanisms for fostering multigenerational resilience. *Contemporary Family Therapy, 36,* 148–161. doi:10.1007/s10591-012-9222-6
Koerin, B. B., & Harrigan, M. P. (2003). P.S. I love you. *Journal of Gerontological Social Work, 40,* 63–81. doi:10.1300/J083v40n01_05
Komarova, N. L., & Thalhauser, C. J. (2011). High degree of heterogeneity in Alzheimer's disease progression patterns. *PLoS Computational Biology, 7,* e1002251. doi:10.1371/journal.pcbi.1002251
Martin, A. S., Distelberg, B. J., & Elahad, J. (2015). The relationship between family resilience and aging successfully. *The American Journal of Family Therapy, 43,* 163–179. doi:10.1080/01926187.2014.988593
Masten, A. S., & Monn, A. R. (2015). Child and family resilience: A call for integrated science, practice, and professional training. *Family Relations, 64,* 5–21. doi:10.1111/fare.12103
McCormick, C. M., Kuo, S. I. C., & Masten, A. S. (2011). Developmental tasks across the lifespan. In K. L. Fingerman, C. A. Berg, J. Smith, & T. C. Antonucci (Eds.), *Handbook of life-span development* (pp. 117–139). New York, NY: Springer.
McCubbin, H. I., & McCubbin, M. A. (1991). Family stress theory and assessment: The resiliency model of family stress, adjustment, and adaptation. In H. I. McCubbin & A. Thompson (Eds.), *Family assessment inventories for research and practice* (pp. 3–21). Madison, WI: University of Wisconsin.
McCubbin, H. I., & Patterson, J. M. (1983). Family transitions: Adaptation to stress. In H. I. McCubbin & C. Figley (Eds.), *Stress and the family: Coping with normative transitions* (pp. 5–25). New York, NY: Brunner/Mazel.
McCubbin, L. D., & McCubbin, H. I. (2013). Resilience in ethnic family systems: A relational theory for research and practice. In D. S. Becvar (Ed.), *Handbook of family resilience* (pp. 175–195). New York, NY: Springer. doi:10.1007/978-1-4614-3917-2_11
McGoldrick, M., & Shibusawa, T.. (2012). The family life cycle. In F. Walsh (Ed.), *Normal family processes: Growing diversity and complexity* (4th ed., pp. 375–398). New York, NY: Guilford.

Moon, M. (2017). The unprepared caregiver. *Gerontologist, 57*(1), 26–31. doi:10.1093/geront/gnw080

Morris, J. C. (1993). Clinical dementia rating (CDR): Current version and scoring rules. *Neurology, 43*, 2412–2414. doi:10.1212/wnl.43.11.2412-a

National Institute of Aging. (2016). *Alzheimer's disease fact sheet.* Retrieved from https://www.nia.nih.gov/alzheimers/publication/alzheimers-disease-fact-sheet#changes

Patterson, J. M. (1988). Families experiencing stress: I. The Family Adjustment and Adaptation Response Model: II. Applying the FAAR model to health related issues for intervention and research. *Family Systems Medicine, 6*, 202–237. doi:10.1037/h0089739

Patterson, J. M. (2002). Integrating family resilience and family stress theory. *Journal of Marriage and the Family, 64*, 349–360. doi:10.1111/j.1741-3737.2002.00349.x

Patterson, J. M., & Garwick, A. W. (1994). Levels of meaning in family stress theory. *Family Process, 33*, 287–304. doi:10.1111/j.1545-5300.1994.00287.x

Qualls, S. H. (this volume). Therapeutic interventions for caregiving families.

Qualls, S. H., & Williams, A. A. (2013). *Caregiver family therapy: Empowering families to meet the challenges of aging.* Washington, DC: American Psychological Association Press.

Reisberg, B. (1988). Functional assessment staging. *Psychopharmacology Bulletin, 4*, 55–659. doi:10.1017/s1041610292001157

Reiss, D. (1981). *The family's construction of reality.* Cambridge: Harvard University Press.

Roberts, E. (this volume). Voices from down home: Family caregiver perspectives on navigating care transitions with individuals with dementia in Nova Scotia, Canada.

Rutter, M. (1987). Psychosocial resilience and protective mechanisms. *American Journal of Orthopsychiatry, 57*, 316–331. doi:10.1111/j.1939-0025.1987.tb03541.x

Rutter, M. (2013). Annual research review: Resilience—Clinical implications. *Journal of Child Psychology and Psychiatry, 54*, 474–487. doi:10.1111/j.1469-7610.2012.02615.x

Sarazin, M., Horne, N., & Dubois, B. (2007). Natural decline and prognostic factors. In S. Gauthier (Ed.), *Clinical diagnosis and management of Alzheimer's disease* (3rd ed., pp. 137–148). London, England: Informa.

Schroder, L. A., & Osteen, S. (this volume). Planning for and managing costs related to caregiving, synthesizing financial planning and gerontology.

Speice, J., Shields, C. G., & Blieszner, R. (1998). The effects of family communication patterns during middle-phase Alzheimer's disease. *Families, Systems & Health, 16*, 233–248. doi:10.1037/h0089852

Taylor, M. G., & Quesnel-Vallée, A. (2017). The structural burden of caregiving: Shared challenges in the United States and Canada. *Gerontologist, 57*(1), 19–25. doi:10.1093/geront/gnw102

Walker, A. J., Pratt, C. C., & Eddy, L. (1995). Informal caregiving to aging family members: A critical review. *Family Relations, 44*, 402–411. http://doi.org/10.2307/584996

Walsh, F. (2012a). Family resilience: Strengths forged through adversity. In F. Walsh (Ed.), *Normal family processes: Growing diversity and complexity* (4th ed., pp. 399–427). New York, NY: Guilford.

Walsh, F. (2012b). Successful aging and family resilience. *Annual Review of Gerontology and Geriatrics, 32*, 151–172. doi:10.1891/0198-8794.32.153

Wright, M. O., Masten, A. S, & Narayan, A. J., (2013). Resilience processes in development: Four waves of research on positive adaptation in the context of adversity. In S. Goldstein & R. B. Brooks (Eds.), *Handbook of resilience in children* (2nd ed., pp. 15–37). New York, NY: Springer. doi:10.1007/978-1-4614-3661-4_2.

Zarit, S. H., Reever, K. E., & Bach-Peterson, J. (1980). Relatives of the impaired elderly: Correlates of feelings of burden. *The Gerontologist, 20*, 649–655. doi:10.1093/geront/20.6.649

Chapter 2
Therapeutic Interventions for Caregiving Families

Sara Honn Qualls

Stories about the challenges, tasks, and relationship transitions related to care for older family members are embedded in daily conversations all around us. Caregiving for older family members has become a normative experience as life expectancy has increased. Most families navigate the challenges well, reporting low rates of burden and distress (Brown & Brown 2014; Roth, Fredman, & Haley, 2015), apparently adapting effectively to the family tasks just as they do at other phases of the family life cycle. Certainly, child-rearing generates plenty of conversation also, because the tasks related to care and rearing of children are compelling, challenging, and at times, distressing. Yet, the normative challenges of childrearing elicit resilience in family structures and processes that are not viewed as inherently problematic. Caregiving for older adults, similarly, can be viewed as a normative family process to which we can anticipate that most families demonstrate resilience, adapting their structures and interpersonal processes to accommodate the unusual needs of one or more older adults.

If providing care is ubiquitous to family life, at what point does it become caregiving? After all, families provide care in patterns that are multi-directional, with reciprocity in giving and receiving care within a brief period of time. Care is provided within generations, between spouses, partners, siblings, and cousins just as it is across generations (AARP & NAC, 2015). Indeed, care might be a defining characteristic of family life. Caregiving occurs when the demands for care cross an often fuzzy line into extraordinary effort and time investment that exceeds what is developmentally expected (Qualls & Williams, 2013). In other words, although families expect short-term care to be reciprocated as needs arise, the chronic and intensive needs for care are those that tax the existing care system (structures and processes) in ways that require substantial adaptation (Aneshensel, Pearlin, Mullan, Zarit, & Whitlatch, 1995). A serious acute illness (e.g., pneumonia, hip fracture) may raise

---

S.H. Qualls, Ph.D. (✉)
University of Colorado Colorado Springs, Psychology Department and Gerontology Center, 4863 Nevada Ave., Suite 350, Colorado Springs, CO 80918, USA
e-mail: squalls@uccs.edu

demands just as chronic diseases such as diabetes, congestive heart failure, or dementia may increase care demands on families (Yorgason et al., 2010).

Viewed through the frame of family resilience, family caregivers are attempting to use familiar family strategies to address what are often novel problems with extended trajectories that can be considered significant risks (Coon, 2012). Counselors and therapists can facilitate family resilience processes across a variety of illnesses, stages of care, situations faced by families, and across diversity in family structure, skills, styles, and cultural contexts (Walsh, 2016). Strategies and frameworks created in the caregiving intervention literature are not yet aligned with those that are taking regular shape in the resilience literature (Henry, Morris, & Harrist, 2015). Common processes that can be used to structure useful family-level therapeutic interventions for caregivers of older adults in this remarkable diversity of circumstances are the focus of this chapter.

This chapter begins with an analysis of the interface of families with healthcare systems, a critical context for the experience of family care for and with older adults. The structure of care over time is then explored as another critical context for understanding what could facilitate family resilience amidst care challenges. Characteristics of successful interventions with particular caregiving populations are then described. Finally, key questions to guide family therapists in helping family caregivers are presented and linked to the family resilience framework.

2.1 The Social Location of Families in Health Care

Caregiving almost universally thrusts families into partnership with professional health care systems, a remarkably fragmented delivery network. Figure 2.1 includes a few of the many systems that support health and well-being, depicting them as disconnected silos with no connective portals.

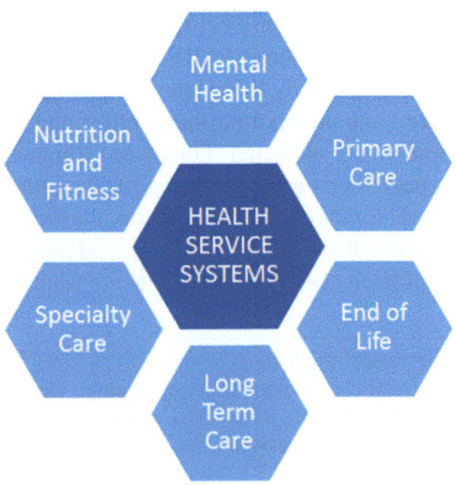

Fig. 2.1 Fragmented health systems faced by families

Almost universally, services are accessed in separate offices whose electronic record systems are rarely connected to other outpatient providers or specialists. Long term care is fully isolated from outpatient or inpatient care systems, without even having internally useful electronic record systems in senior housing or most assisted living facilities. End of life care is viewed as discontinuous with other health systems that focus on cure. The nutrition and fitness industries are promoting health and well-being in nearly complete isolation from other health systems. Mental health services are now integrating into primary care, but rarely in the other service systems where older adults access services (e.g., social services, housing). The costs to human life and quality of life have been documented by the Institute of Medicine who defines the systems as broken enough to need a substantial overhaul (U.S. Institute of Medicine, 2001).

Families face the challenges of meeting the needs of members within these disconnected systems, with nearly full responsibility placed on individuals and their families for transitioning across them. For each of the multiple care episodes that will occur across a lifespan, the family is the social and cultural unit that is expected by the formal care systems (e.g., health, social services) to "own" health and care during the episode and across the transitions, especially for frail or cognitively compromised older members. Labeled as the *caregiver assumption*, this phenomenon has shared cultural buy-in that is embedded in public policies (Bailey & Gordon, 2016).

The family lacks a place on the health system organizational chart, reflecting the absence of a clear role for family in healthcare. Family roles that are documented in health records include that of collateral informant at the point of entry into services and proxy decision-maker. Occasionally, family is required to be with a patient after a medical procedure. However, families are ignored routinely as health partners who have a heavy investment in information gathering, tracking, implementation of treatments, and who share in (and constrain) health behavior patterns that are critical to preventing or managing chronic disease (McDaniel, Doherty, & Hepworth, 2013). Families often notice critical signs of changes in health status long before more blatant symptoms emerge that would be recognized by a provider who lacks the intimate familiarity within family life. Changes in diet, physical activity, medication administration, or treatment implementation are likely to affect family members' activities, and thus can serve as deterrents for self-management of health and disease. Yet health systems lack a coordinated way in which to recognize the roles of families in the ongoing health and wellness of its consumers. Even the emerging model for a medical home in which primary care serves a centralized organizing function lacks a place for family interface.

Families vary in the roles they allocate to health systems. Consider two very different models for family interface with health systems depicted in Fig. 2.2.

The left side illustrates an individualistic model in which each component of the health system interfaces with the patient separately without any contact with the family except through the patient. The right side illustrates a very different model in which patients view themselves as embedded in their families who live within cultural contexts of support and services. The latter model can generate conflicts within a health system that wants to communicate only with the patient, yet expects full family support for care when needed (e.g., at discharge from one service, or as informant during entrance into a service system). Add long term care to the picture, and families are obviously likely to be confused by the incongruent expectations for their participation that one system establishes as full responsibility while another system experiences participation as intrusive or interruptive of their jobs.

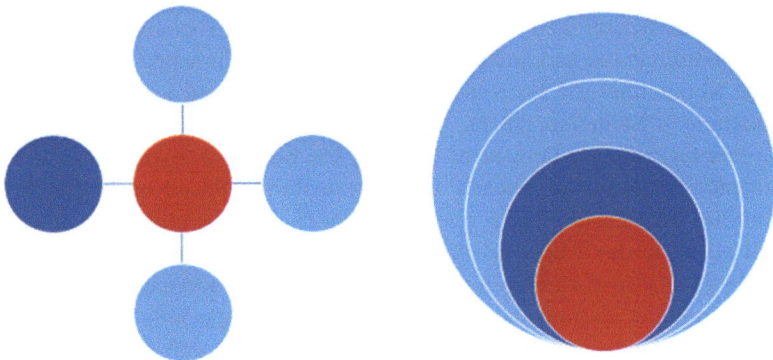

Fig. 2.2 Two models of family position with patients and health service systems

---

Breakout Box 2.1 Focus on Interdisciplinary Work
I have had many experiences with caregiving on both a personal and professional level. Over the years, I have identified key factors of both family caregivers and health care providers that create the most successful environment. The most critical of these factors is providing patient centered care, in which multiple facets of patient's care system are integrated. Information sharing by all parties involved assists with getting everyone on the same page and eliminates possible stressors that are inevitable when there are gaps in a patient's care system. A patient's care system could include attending physicians, home health care providers, nurses, dietitians, mental health providers, extended family, and other social support. While some regulatory guidelines could limit collaboration, there are major advantages for patients' health and safety when these components are allowed to do integrative work.

Family members in a caregiving role assume an important position in that they have the greatest understanding of the patient prior to and following the onset illness/disability. Incorporating this information into treatment plans is valuable to patient's resilience, and requires family members to be involved, present, and open to developing relationship with varies members of the healthcare system. One important way family members can be involved is by

(continued)

> **Box 2.1** (continued)
> asking questions to gain a greater understanding of what they are dealing with and options they have. Another key factor in promoting resilience in caregiving families is clearly defining roles and expectations in such a way that the caregiving load is distributed throughout multiple willing and able members. Being a family member in a caregiving role can create difficulties not only emotionally and physically, but also by placing strains on the caregiver's additional roles and finances. A solution to this strain is participating in guilt-free respite time to step out of a caregiver role allowing caregivers the chance to rejuvenate and minimize the possibility of burnout. Minimizing caregiving burnout helps ensure the best care for patients. From all aspects, resilience is best achieved when the patient is surrounded by supportive caregivers who are both willing and able to accurately advocate for the patients best interest.
> —Maria Avers, RN, FCN, MSNE, Director of Stillwater Medical Center Home Health.

2.2 Family Care Trajectories

Chronic diseases are experienced over long periods of time, with shifts in the needs for family care services as the disease progresses (Rolland, 2012). Figure 2.3 illustrates the transitions that families experience as care needs change over the course of the illness (Qualls & Williams, 2013, p. 26).

When the disease begins, the family has structures and processes in place that are not organized around caregiving. At some point, the illness becomes sufficiently visible or salient that the family needs to, and usually does, adapt its familiar processes and structures to accommodate caregiving. In the case of illnesses that produce dementias, or progressive cognitive impairments, the early caregiving adaptations focus on shifting strategies for accomplishing Instrumental Activities of Daily Living (IADLs), those activities that support independent living in the community (e.g., medication management, transportation, shopping). Progression of the disease leads the family into accommodating needs for assistance with basic Activities of Daily Living (ADLs) such as bathing, toileting, dressing, transferring, mobility, and feeding. For many chronic physical illnesses or disabilities, progression of functional impairment can compromise autonomous completion of ADLs before IADL autonomy is affected. Loss of sensory functioning (e.g., hearing, vision) or mobility may constrain a person's ability to accomplish basic self-care independently even when their cognitive abilities needed to organize and maintain IADL functioning is fully intact (Yorgason et al., 2010). In sum, family caregiving roles are shaped by the trajectory of functional decline that the illness imposes on the care recipient. Over time, those roles change as self-care abilities decline.

Families often ask health providers to project the rate and slope of the trajectory of declining functioning for a particular illness. Their questions often take the form

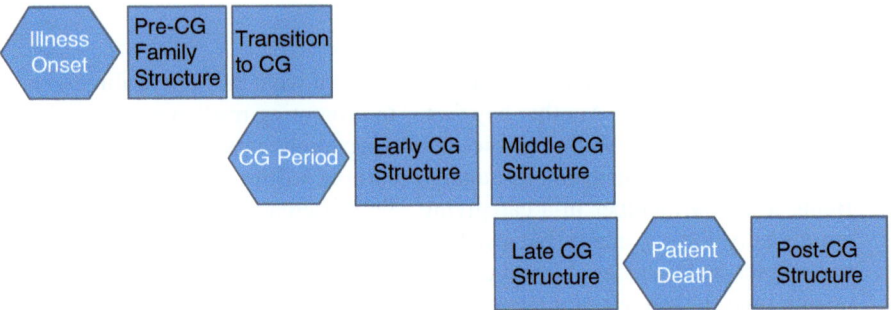

Fig. 2.3 Caregiving stages. From Qualls and Williams (2013, p. 26), used with permission

of "How will we know when it is time to …?" or "How long until we need to add x service?". Unfortunately, this type of information that seems so critical to families is difficult for health providers to supply, and thus less comfortable for them to discuss than diagnostic evaluations or treatment plans. Trajectories of functional decline due to chronic disease are quite variable across individuals is due to many factors, including genetics, medical co-morbidities, environmental support, and other idiosyncratic factors (Gabriel, 2011). Probabilistic statements based on population data are of limited value to projecting the course for a particular person. Furthermore, almost all conditions generate significant intra-individual variability over time and those with the disease experience major shifts in functioning upward and downward over time. Some diseases produce hour by hour variations in care needs whereas others show fluctuations over the course of days, months, or years. Many families learn to expect interruptions in health functioning, periods when an illness draws down the energy needed to function in the existing environment. This intra-individual variability can demand extraordinary flexibility from families, who must approach each day as an experiment in what type of role support is needed on that day or hour. Of course, families vary in the levels of resources available within their adaptive system prior to the onset of the illness, and thus vary in the successful activation of stress response systems to the demands of illness(es) (Henry et al., 2015).

2.3 Help-Seeking by Families

Relatively little is known about caregiver help-seeking generally and even less for particular populations. Variations are influenced by sociocultural factors such as economic and social resources, ethnicity and race, geography, and a myriad of factors that influence the ways in which problems are conceptualized and addressed, and the ways in which families experience stress and burden (Knight & Sayengh, 2010).

Assistance for family caregivers is available from a wide range of sources. The Older Americans Act (2000) authorizes and funds services for caregivers of persons age 60 and over as well as older adults caring for persons under age 18. Funds are distributed from the federal government to states who typically distribute them through the Area Agencies on Aging (AAA) that operate at the local level. Included in caregiver services funding are outreach activities to distribute information about caregiving to the public, respite care, and counseling. Some caregivers go to caregiving workshops, pampering days, or outreach fairs where considerable information and support can be accessed in a short period of time. Others seek individual counseling from these funded services or other resources in the health and human services networks. Attorneys and health providers also provide support for family caregivers of older adults, but often with a focus on caregivers' experiences secondary to the focus on care recipients. Caregivers' needs are rarely assessed directly or comprehensively. Faith communities are increasing their focus on health promotion and support for frail individuals, activities that lead them into increasing awareness of the needs of caregivers.

Unfortunately, the timing of access to information about social services is at least as tricky as is access to appropriate health care. Families often have difficulty connecting with useful resources in a timely manner, and when resources are needed in multiple domains, the probability of getting the resources all aligned seems quite low. When a loved one's health declines, family caregivers find themselves scrambling to address rapidly changing needs with appropriate responses and resources. As with all stages of family life, we tend to seek help on a need-to-know basis so we face the challenges of the next stage of family life without the requisite knowledge or skills. We rarely educate ourselves about the stages of the family life cycle that lie ahead of us. Parents of pre-schoolers are unlikely to invest significant time trying to understand the challenges and opportunities of life in family with adolescents. Similarly, the tasks of family life with frail older adults appear rather suddenly in our lives, without knowledge, skills, or experience to prepare us. Perhaps even more in social services than in healthcare, families often struggle to figure out what they need, and where to find it.

Families often delay the identification of health problems that present themselves in ways that can easily be attributed to normal aging, personality, or other non-medical causes seem likely to delay help-seeking. Caregivers of persons with dementia describe delaying medical evaluation for a year or more, during which behavior problems were observed prior to the evaluation that led to diagnosis (Knopman, Donahue, & Gutterman, 2000). Furthermore, multiple provocative events that threaten the safety of the loved one are, together, the trigger that prompted action to seek the evaluation (Nichols & Martindale-Adams, 2006; Streams, Wackerbarth, & Maxwell, 2003. Models of medical help-seeking have emphasized the importance of risk appraisals as a factor that provokes help-seeking, along with the cognitive schema through which the family member observes changes that are understood as related to medical problems (Qualls et al., 2015). In short, families seek help when they are worried. Caregivers seek assistance from a broad array of providers because building knowledge and skill about where to find resources is a part of their journey. Understanding family help-seeking patterns will help providers assist the family effectively.

2.4 Successful Interventions with Family Caregivers

Interventions to reduce burden and distress in caregivers have been developed and tested for many caregiving populations in the past 30 years since the topic garnered substantial national attention. Although caregivers for persons with dementia have been the focus of the largest number of intervention studies, benefits among caregivers of persons with other diseases have resulted from interventions as well (Burgio, Gaugler, & Hilgeman, 2016; Coon, Keaveny, Valverde, Dadvar, & Gallagher-Thompson, 2012).

Common factors characterize successful interventions as well as disease or condition-specific components to the interventions (Pinquart & Sörensen, 2006). Almost all interventions include information sharing, most often at the level of broad information about the care recipient's disease or condition or common experiences of caregivers. Almost all interventions provide information in multiple modalities, often combining written or online handouts that can be reviewed at home with oral presentations that interpret and apply the information. Successful interventions with caregivers tend to be active, adding to empathy some form of explicit action-orientation for the caregiver to use (Burgio & Gaugler, 2016). The focus varies across interventions, such that the action may be targeted at one of two things: changing the frequency and type of self-care by the caregiver or changing strategies for addressing challenges presented by a care recipient's illness or condition. Most interventions engage in some form of problem-solving, whether focused on meeting the needs of the care recipient or the caregiver.

Enhancements of social support for the caregiver are also an explicit focus of many efficacious interventions (e.g., Belle et al., 2006; Mittelman, Ferris, Shulman, Steinberg, & Levin, 1996). Feelings of burden and isolation tend to decrease when the frequency, intensity, or focus of social support improves the caregiver's perception of support (Burgio & Gaugler, 2016; Pinquart & Sörensen, 2006).

Successful interventions link caregiving families with resources in their communities to extend and expand the options for meeting the needs of care recipients and caregivers. Families may be referred to health providers with specialty in the care recipients' conditions, respite care, in-home services, residential alternatives, and/or legal counsel that can advise on appropriate legal decision-making structures. Most families are introduced to the AAA network of providers across the country that serve offer comprehensive information on local resources along with caregiver support services (find local AAA at www.eldercare.gov). Care recipients' illnesses may be the focus of a consumer-support organization where information and support groups specific to that condition are available (e.g., Alzheimer's disease, Parkinson's disease, or depression).

The literature on interventions is quite limited, despite the fact that many interventions exist to assist caregiving families (Burgio & Gaugler, 2016). The vast majority of studies examine an approach that was developed and tested with specific populations in mind (e.g., dementia, stroke), thus limiting generalizability. Furthermore, the samples recruited for clinical trials are likely to differ substantially from those who seek help in more naturalistic ways within a community, thus raising questions about how the interventions may need to be adapted for other types of families who are not represented in those studies (Zarit & Femia, 2008). The evidence base for interventions varies significantly across populations and strategies, with a small subset having been tested in enough rigorous trials to be recognized as evidence-based interventions within the Registry managed by the Substance Abuse and Mental Health Services Administration (Substance Abuse and Mental Health Services Administration, n.d.; available at http://www.samhsa.gov/nrepp). The vast majority of interventions have a research base that is too small or that uses methodologies not recognized by the Registry. Furthermore, dissemination research on the impact of those interventions when implemented outside of a research setting is quite weak (Burgio & Gaugler, 2016).

Another limitation is that the "active ingredients" in the interventions are not yet determined through empirical testing (Burgio & Gaugler, 2016). The push to tailor or individualize interventions for particular families will rely increasingly on an understanding of the active ingredients as providers design interventions that target the particular needs of particular families dealing with particular problems using a *dose* or amount of intervention designed to match the intensity of the need. Tailoring interventions will be facilitated by comprehensive approaches to caregiving challenges that offer decision points for shaping the intervention for a particular caregiver or family.

2.5 Implications for Practice: Caregiver Family Therapy, a Framework to Guide Interventions with Caregiving Families

While caregiving approaches have been developed and tested for particular populations, an approach was evolving in a clinic setting that counsels caregivers for older adults with a wide variety of illnesses and needs. This approach conceptualizes families as the primary social context for interventions, and thus frames the model as a family therapy model called Caregiver Family Therapy (CFT), expanding what can be provided and for whom within an intervention.

The CFT approach is designed to guide counselors or other providers in work with a broad range of caregiving family members addressing a broad range of problems in the caregiver, care recipient, or the caregiving circumstance, including the family system. CFT *assists families with recognizing, interpreting, and taking action to address age-related problems while continuing to meet the needs of multiple family members* (Qualls & Williams, 2013). By offering a systematic sequence of questions to be addressed by the provider and client, the intervention can be tailored to meet particular needs. The familial context of care, both giving and receiving, is an explicit framework for this approach.

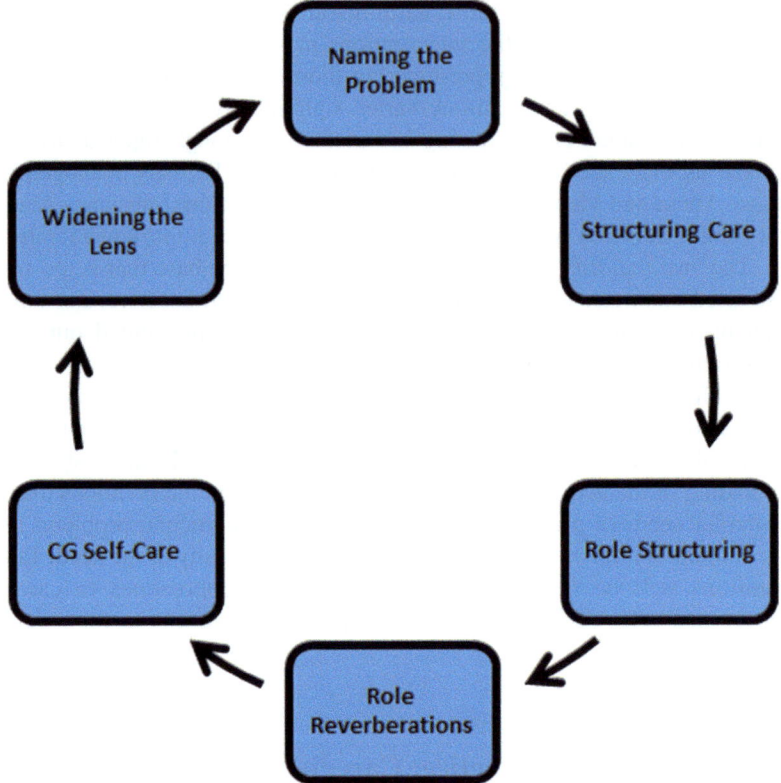

Fig. 2.4 Caregiver family therapy components. Adapted from Qualls and Williams (2013, p. 7), used with permission

The six domains in the CFT model focus providers on the core components of the family system's care structure that can facilitate resilience, thus leading to a stable approach to providing care that allows the family to function effectively for many family members (see Fig. 2.4). The intervention with one family may need to address the Naming the Problem, Care Structure, and Role Structure components first whereas another family may have a strong understanding of the problem and a working care structure, but serious problems with negotiating useful and sustainable Role Structures, dealing with Role Reverberations, and caregiver Self-Care.

2.5.1 Naming the Problem

Once a family caregiver reaches out for help, providers need a systematic way to assess the problems that are described. Families describe their caregiving experiences, including the care recipients' experiences of illness, using language familiar to them that is often quite different language than that used by providers. Thus, providers who encounter families of older adults need to appreciate the diverse phrases and names used to describe changes in the biopsychosocial functioning of older adults. "He's stubborn" may be used to describe a lifelong personality trait that contributed to career success but is now more difficult to manage at home, or may describe resistance to self-care that reflects diminished cognitive ability to initiate and follow instructions. "She can do so much more than she will do—she's just not motivated." "He used to walk the dog every day, now he just sits—he's so depressed." "She hates it when I help her—she always cries or gets mad." "She won't plan ahead for bathrooming, and inevitably gets in trouble in the middle of a store." All of these descriptors are loaded with rich information about the functioning of the caregiver and care recipient, but cannot be assumed to be accurate in diagnosis of the source of the problem. What may appear as low motivation as part of depression, could be cognitive difficulties with initiation due to a brain disease or nutritional deficits that produce delirium. Careful assessment of the care recipient is often key to helping the caregiver develop an accurate understanding of strengths and challenges faced by care recipients. CFT therapists sometimes conduct that assessment, but more often are able to gather materials from others' assessments or refer for additional evaluation so sufficient information is available to assist the family in developing a shared understanding of the care recipient's situation that is accurate.

2.5.2 Care Structure

Caregivers may present their request for help as a question about resource availability. "Where is the best assisted living facility in my part of town?" "Which memory care units take Medicaid?" "Which neurologists take Medicare?" These questions can and should be answered. However, in the ideal scenario, the source of the information will also query the caregiver about the situation in order to see if there are other questions that might be relevant. For example, how does a family decide that assisted living is the right level of support for a particular person? Families often begin their search for support using the frame and knowledge they have as they enter this phase of the family life cycle. A particular family may have appraised the care recipient to be at risk in his or her current situation, and begin to investigate strategies for reducing risk by looking into housing options. This family might be inaccurate in its assessment of risk, having simply responded to observing that the care recipient is different from previous years. Additionally, the family may be unaware of many community supports that might reduce risk in the current living situation. Thus, the request for information about residential options may have been their first stop in the process of information gathering, during which a savvy provider can help them open their investigation to a broader set of questions that will lead to resources that could never have been requested by the family due to ignorance that they existed.

A common help-seeking question for families is about how to time transitions in levels of support. *How do I know when it is time to get her more services.... To help her move into a smaller place.... To take the car keys... To take over management of her bills or medications... To help him move back home like he wants to do?* The timing of these transitions is dependent upon a range of factors, including values and preferences of the care recipient and caregiver, but also on objective functional information about capabilities and risk, trajectories of illnesses, and availability of various types of resources. In other words, the picture is complex, and the family is struggling with its appraisal of risk and safety. Interventions usually include the sharing of information about resources that can educate, guide, or partner with families in providing appropriate care for the care recipient.

2.5.3 Role Structure

Even in families that have obtained a clear understanding of the problem and appropriate care structures, the question of *how* to implement those care structures can impede action. Families realize that some of these actions require them to take on new roles that represent quite significant changes in the relationship. *He hasn't seen a doctor in 20 years, and he's not going to agree to go now. She won't agree to quit driving without a fight. He won't move anywhere—he insists on staying in his home until he dies.* These statements are part of a plea to help the speaker figure out how to accomplish the task. They also reflect particular role structures in the family that constrain the speaker from a range of actions that might be possible if the roles were to change. Not unlike the perplexed parent of a teenager who has reached the limits of persuasion to change behavior, a caregiver may need assistance figuring out small or large role shifts that open the door to alternative ways of interacting that may be more productive to accomplish the behavior change. In the case of later life families, those role changes represent very significant departures from previous definitions of roles such as wife/husband, daughter/son, or sister/brother.

Families have many ways that they can organize care for a member who requires assistance. One person may be recognized as the primary caregiver, with others serving support roles or abdicating contribution to care. Alternatively, two or more persons may share the primary care roles. Roles may be strongly prescribed, as occurs in families that expect the oldest son or oldest daughter to be responsible for care. In other families, the selection is shaped by pragmatics such as who lives nearby, who has the skills to provide particular services (e.g., medical or financial), or by personality. Research suggests that the key is having a defined structure related to decision-making so the family is clear about who has authority to make what decisions (Lieberman & Fisher, 1999). Full democracy seems to work no better in later life families than it does during child-rearing. At least child-rearing families have clear identification of the decision-making authority with parents at least until late adolescence or early adulthood, but later life families often have to be more explicit in identifying whom to sanction with what authority, and how to implement the communication around roles.

2.5.4 Role Reverberations

Once a family member accepts caregiving responsibilities in any form (primary or support), the caregiver usually experiences some impact of this role on other roles. Reverberations of the caregiving role are often apparent in other family relationships and roles. One's roles as spouse, parent, sibling, or child are likely to be affected as caregiving demands have an impact on available time, effort, energy, and creativity. Friendships, community roles, and employment are also likely to be affected by the caregiving role. In some cases, family caregivers have structured care in a way that fit the values and preferences of caregiver or care recipient, but without counting the cost to other roles. For example, a daughter may drive across town early each morning to bathe, dress, and prepare breakfast for her mother prior to going to her job as a bank executive. The evening routine may involve preparing dinner, sharing the evening meal to ensure mother eats well, and preparing mother for bed. Although this pattern may fit the expectations and values of mother and daughter, it is likely to have a substantial impact on the daughter's work performance over time, as well as her spouse, parenting, and friend roles. An additional role reverberation occurs within the relationship between caregiver and care recipient. Caregiving often unbalances the historic give and take within the relationship, a challenge to all aspects of the relationship dynamics, meaning, and even dignity. Examining the reverberations of caregiving roles on other roles invites the caregiver to look at how particular care patterns impact the broad structures of her life and well-being.

2.5.5 Self-Care

The extraordinary demands of chronic care can easily undermine the caregiver's consistency in caring for her own needs. Indeed, self-care may appear to a caregiver as a selfish concern in the face of the importance of meeting the care recipient's needs, particularly if the care recipient is quite vulnerable. CFT positions the self-care topic at this point in the intervention to ensure that the caregiver has indeed structured an effective and appropriate system of care that can be sustained. When self-care is introduced early in an intervention, caregivers can readily discount its importance in the face of urgent issues related to safety or quality of life for the care recipient. Unless self-neglect has put the caregiver in a health crisis that demands immediate intervention, CFT waits to address self-care until the roles are structured to meet the needs of the care recipient while accommodating the caregiver's other roles.

A biopsychosocial framework for well-being suggests that self-care needs to address multiple domains of well-being for caregivers. Nutrition, exercise, regular physical examinations, adherence to recommended medical treatments, and sufficient sleep are common biological self-care challenges for caregivers. Psychological self-care may include self-efficacy to handle caregiving tasks, perceived control and mastery over a range of life domains in addition to caregiving, and time and frameworks to grieve losses in functioning of the care recipient and the relationship. Social relationships can be starved by the demands of caregiving, or new relationships may add new opportunities and demands that require some thoughtful effort. In short, caregivers need to adapt a range of self-care strategies that have worked in the past to be sustainable during the caregiving period. They may also need to develop new strategies to enhance self-care beyond previous levels due to the extraordinary demands of caregiving.

2.5.6 Widening the Lens

The final step in an episode of CFT is to widen the lens to look at the bigger picture, to examine how caregiving structures are affecting the well-being of the family as a whole, and how caregiving may unfold over time. As an intervention nears closure for the episode at hand, caregivers can be invited to step back to look at the wider impact of caregiving on the family. Who may be affected indirectly by the care structures? If the caregiver is providing care to one member, are there other members who have lost support, guidance, or other aspects of a relationship with the caregiver? Whereas the role reverberation examined the caregiver's role performance across a range of family relationships, the lens is now widened to look at the family's investments in caregiving from the vantage point of other members. The key question is whether every member's developmental needs are being met within the current structures at least as well as they were prior to the intrusion of caregiving demands. A spouse caregiver may recognize that she has less time and attention for a grandchild with special needs during the period when she needs to invest heavily in her husband's care. With this awareness, she may be able to discuss this gap in support for this grandchild with other family members who can increase their rate of engagement so the grandchild is not adversely affected by caregiving to the grandfather.

Looking ahead to anticipate changes in care needs is the other aspect of widening the lens that occurs near the end of an intervention. Most caregiving situations can be anticipated to change as the care recipient's illness or condition changes over time. Most chronic diseases have trajectories of decline that are not simple to predict in timing, but the decline in functioning, pain, or symptoms is relatively predictable. CFT encourages caregivers to picture what changes might alter the stability of the current care structure. What might be signs that the care recipient is changing or the caregiver is burning out? What resources may be useful in the future? What cues would indicate that the family might benefit from re-thinking the strategies in place, additional support, or counseling? One goal of this step is to normalize change so families can anticipate that adaptation will be ongoing. Another is to note how caregiving has a broad reach into the family structure, and to be creative in how to ensure that all members' needs are met even while one member has extraordinary need.

In summary, CFT is intended to be useful for caregivers at any stage of care for persons dealing with a wide variety of conditions that warrant supportive care. The approach is an umbrella framework for identifying the particular needs that the family is struggling to address using their families adaptation strategies. Within this framework, many existing evidence-based approaches can be incorporated as effective strategies. The steps or components are intended to be asked sequentially, but the intervention rarely follows a particular sequence. Instead, care structuring may lead the caregiver back to clarify how to name some aspect of the problem, or self-care interventions may lead a caregiver to re-visit the structure of care or the caregiving roles.

2.6 Conclusion

As the backbone of healthcare for older adults in the U.S., family caregiving resilience is critical to the diverse tasks, structures, and trajectories of care. Most families demonstrate remarkable resilience in caregiving processes, despite a clear lack of integration of their roles and activities into the formal healthcare system. This chapter examined some challenges faced by families, and offered a brief summary of approaches to intervening to support resilient responses to caregiving. The caregiver family therapy model focuses on key questions to guide family therapists in helping family caregivers and links well to the family resilience framework.

Questions for Thought and Discussion

1. Think about how each of the Family Adaptive Systems (FAS) proposed in Henry et al. (2015)—emotion systems, control systems, meaning systems, maintenance systems, and family stress response systems—might play a role in the resilience of a family facing caregiving challenges when working with the health care and social services.
2. How do the FAS interface with the caregiver family therapy components outlined by Qualls?
3. Qualls points out that the challenges of caring for a young child are normalized in modern society: "…the normative challenges of childrearing elicit resilience in family structures and processes that are not viewed as inherently problematic"—yet caregiving for older adults does not seem to have become normalized in the same way. What might change this?
4. Recent studies (e.g., Whitebird et al., 2013) have shown that mindfulness-based stress reduction can be effective for family caregivers. If you were working with a support group of caregivers and introduced the idea of daily mindfulness practices and group members resisted because they were too busy, how would you respond?

References

AARP, & National Alliance for Caregiving. (2015). *Caregiving in the U.S. 2015*. National Alliance for Caregiving and American Association of Retired Persons. Retrieved from http://www.caregiving.org/wp-content/uploads/2015/05/2015_CaregivingintheUS_Final-Report-June-4_WEB.pdf

Aneshensel, C. S., Pearlin, L. I., Mullan, J. T., Zarit, S. H., & Whitlatch, C. J. (1995). *Profiles in caregiving: The unexpected career*. San Diego, CA: Academic Press.

Bailey, W. A., & Gordon, S. R. (2016). Family caregiving amidst age-associated cognitive changes: Implications for practice and future generations. *Family Relations, 65*, 225–238. doi:10.1111/fare.12176

Belle, S. H., Burgio, L., Burns, R., Coon, D., Czaja, S. J., Gallagher-Thompson, D., ... Martindal-Adams, J. (2006). Enhancing the quality of life of dementia caregivers from different ethnic or racial groups. *Annals of Internal Medicine, 145*, 727–738. doi:10.7326/0003-4819-145-10-200611210-00005

Brown, R. M., & Brown, S. L. (2014). Informal caregiving: A reappraisal of effects on caregivers. *Social Issues and Policy Review, 8*, 74–102. doi:10.1111/sipr.12002

Burgio, L. D., & Gaugler, J. E. (2016). Caregiving for the chronically ill: State of the science and future directions. In L. D. Burgio, J. E. Gaugler, & M. M. Hilgeman (Eds.), *The spectrum of family caregiving for adults and elders with chronic illness* (pp. 258–278). New York, NY: Oxford University Press.

Burgio, L. D., Gaugler, J. E., & Hilgeman, M. M. (2016). *The spectrum of family caregiving for adults and elders with chronic illness*. New York, NY: Oxford University Press.

Coon, D. W. (2012). Resilience and family caregiving. In B. J. Hayslip, G. C. Smith, B. J. Hayslip, & G. C. Smith (Eds.), *Annual review of gerontology and geriatrics, Vol 32: Emerging perspectives on resilience in adulthood and later life* (pp. 231–249). New York, NY: Springer.

Coon, D. W., Keaveny, M., Valverde, I. R., Dadvar, S., & Gallagher-Thompson, D. (2012). Evidence-based psychological treatments for distress in family caregivers of older adults. In F. Scogin & A. Shah (Eds.), *Making evidence-based psychological treatments work with older adults* (pp. 225–284). Washington, DC: APA Press.

Gabriel, M. S. (2011). Trajectories of chronic illness. In S. H. Qualls & J. E. Kasl-Godley (Eds.), *End-of-life issues, grief, and bereavement* (pp. 26–42). Hoboken, NJ: Wiley.

Henry, C. S., Morris, A. S., & Harrist, A. W. (2015). Family resilience: Moving into the third wave. *Family Relations, 64*, 22–43. doi:10.1111/fare.12106

Knight, B. G., & Sayengh, P. (2010). Cultural values and caregiving: The updated sociocultural stress and coping model. *Journals of Gerontology: Series B: Psychological Sciences, 65B*, 5–13. doi:10.1093/geronb/gbp096

Knopman, D., Donahue, J. A., & Gutterman, E. M. (2000). Patterns of care in the early stages of Alzheimer's disease: Impediments to timely diagnosis. *Journal of the American Geriatrics Society, 48*, 300–304. doi:10.1111/j.1532-5415.2000.tb02650.x

Lieberman, M. A., & Fisher, L. (1999). The effects of family conflict resolution and decision making on the provision of help for an elder with Alzheimer's disease. *Gerontologist, 39*, 159–166. doi:10.1093/geront/39.2.159

McDaniel, S. H., Doherty, W., & Hepworth, J. (2013). *Medical family therapy and integrated care* (2nd ed.). Washington, DC: American Psychological Association.

Mittelman, M. S., Ferris, S. H., Shulman, E., Steinberg, G., & Levin, B. (1996). A family intervention to delay nursing home placement of patients with Alzheimer disease. *JAMA, 276*, 1725–1731. doi:10.1001/jama.1996.03540210033030

Nichols, L. O., & Martindale-Adams, J. (2006). The decisive moment: Caregivers' recognition of dementia. *Clinical Gerontologist, 30*, 39–52. doi:10.1300/J018v30n01_04

Older Americans Act Amendments of 2000. (2000). Title III Section 316. *National Family Caregiver Support Program*. U.S.C. 3030s.

Pinquart, M., & Sörensen, S. (2006). Helping caregivers of persons with dementia: Which interventions work and how large are their effects? *International Psychogeriatrics, 18*, 577–595. doi:10.1017/S1041610206003462

Qualls, S. H., Klebe, K. J., Berryman, K., Williams, A., Phillips, L., Layton, H., ... Rogers, M. (2015). Motivational and cognitive pathways to medical help-seeking for Alzheimer's disease: A cognitive impairment response model. *The Journals of Gerontology: Psychological Sciences, 70*, 57–66. doi:10.1093/geronb/gbu058

Qualls, S. H., & Williams, A. A. (2013). *Caregiver family therapy*. Washington, DC: APA Press.
Rolland, J. S. (2012). Mastering family challenges in serious illness and disability. In F. Walsh (Ed.), *Normal family processes* (4th ed.pp. 452–482). New York, NY: Guilford.
Roth, D. L., Fredman, L., & Haley, W. E. (2015). Informal caregiving and its impact on health: A reappraisal from population-based studies. *The Gerontologist, 55*, 309–319. doi:10.1093/geront/gnu177
Streams, M. E., Wackerbarth, S. B., & Maxwell, A. (2003). Diagnosis-seeking at subspecialty memory clinics: Trigger events. *International Journal of Geriatric Psychiatry, 18*, 915–924. doi:10.1002/gps.946
Substance Abuse and Mental Health Services Administration. (n.d.). *National registry of evidence-based programs and practices*. Retrieved from http://www.samhsa.gov/nrepp
U.S. Institute of Medicine. (2001). *Crossing the quality chasm: A new health system for the 21st century*. doi:10.17226/10027.
Walsh, F. (2016). *Strengthening family resilience* (3rd ed.). New York, NY: Guilford Press.
Whitebird, R. R., Kreitzer, M., Crain, A. L., Lewis, B. A., Hanson, L. R., & Enstad, C. J. (2013). Mindfulness-based stress reduction for family caregivers: A randomized controlled trial. *The Gerontologist, 53*, 676–686. doi:10.1093/geront/gns126
Yorgason, J. B., Roper, S. O., Wheeler, B., Crane, K., Byron, R., Carpenter, L., ... Higley, D. (2010). Older couples' management of multiple-chronic illnesses: Individual and shared perceptions and coping in type 2 diabetes and osteoarthritis. *Families, Systems, & Health, 28*, 30–47. doi:10.1037/a0019396
Zarit, S. H., & Femia, E. E. (2008). A future for family care and dementia intervention research? Challenges and strategies. *Aging & Mental Health, 12*, 5–13. doi:10.1080/13607860701616317

Chapter 3
Resilience Through Nutrition: Nutritional and Dietary Challenges and Opportunities for Caregiving Families

Janice R. Hermann and Kristopher M. Struckmeyer

With one in five Americans expected to be age 65 years or over by 2030 (Kendall, Hillers, & Medeiros, 2006), a public health crisis is beginning to ensue. Increased longevity has been linked to increases in disability and functional dependency prevalence in older adults (Silver & Wellman, 2002). Functional limitations can impact older adults' ability to grocery shop and prepare meals; affecting food intake (Hermann, Brosi, Johnston, & Jaco, 2012). Poor nutrition is a frequent condition amongst older adults (Rullier et al., 2014), creating a possible downward spiral of decline. Nutritional well-being contributes to better health and self-sufficiency, as well as promoting quality of life (American Dietetic Association [ADA], 2000; Hermann et al., 2012), yet older adults who cannot obtain proper nutrition are at risk for functional changes related to poor nutrition (Amarantos, Martinez, & Dwyer, 2001), increasing their risk for malnutrition and further decreased functional ability; resulting in increased dependence on others for grocery shopping and meal preparation (Hermann et al., 2012). As of 2015, 76% of caregivers help their care recipients with grocery shopping, while 61% report assisting with meal preparation (National Alliance on Caregiving & AARP Public Policy Institute, 2015). These findings show that caregivers have a critical role in helping their care recipients obtain a healthful diet.

Several studies (e.g., Rullier, Lagarde, Bouisson, Bergua, & Barberger-Gateau, 2013; Rullier et al., 2014) have noted that the care recipient's nutritional status is linked to the nutritional status of the caregiver. Poorer health outcomes for caregiv-

---

J.R. Hermann, Ph.D., R.D./L.D. (✉)
Department of Nutritional Sciences, 308 Human Sciences, Oklahoma State University, Stillwater, OK 74078, USA
e-mail: janice.hermann@okstate.edu

K.M. Struckmeyer, M.S.
Department of Human Development & Family Science, Oklahoma State University, Stillwater, OK, USA
e-mail: struckm@okstate.edu

ers are related to poorer health outcomes for care recipients, as well as diminished involvement in self-care promotion (e.g., regular exercise, good nutrition, and stress management) (Castro et al., 2007). Acton (2002) defines health promoting self-care as actions individuals take to "improve their health, maintain optimal functioning, and increase general well-being" (p. 73). Acton further explains that these actions, while possibly in response to illness symptoms, are primarily used to promote health in the absence of illness symptoms. Engaging in health-promoting behaviors (e.g., proper nutrition and exercise) can moderate the effects of stress and decrease morbidity and mortality risks (Ross, Sundaramurthi, & Bevans, 2013). However, caregivers are less likely to engage in self-care activities, such as regular exercise or proper nutrition (Castro et al., 2007) due to high levels of stress. Caregivers who report high stress levels are more susceptible to self-medicating with alcohol, drugs, and fattening foods (Ross et al., 2013).

3.1 Nutritional Problems in Caregiving Families

Despite widespread awareness of what constitutes healthy eating, incidences of diet-related chronic illnesses continue to rise, indicative of poor application of appropriate nutrition knowledge (Hollywood et al., 2013). Thornton, Jeffery, and Crawford (2012) note that healthy behaviors are influenced by an individual's ability to make healthy choices, his/her motivation to make those choices, and the environmental opportunities present to make those choices. When asked about barriers to healthy eating, caregivers cited low confidence in ability to shop, prep, or cook healthy foods (Hollywood et al., 2013; Stead, Caraher, & Anderon, 2004; Thornton et al., 2012), misconceptions about appropriate nutrition for older adults (Watkinson-Powell, Barnes, Lovatt, Wasielewska, & Drummond, 2014), cost and access to healthy foods (Barre, Ferron, Davis, & Whitley, 2011), and less family support for healthier eating (Thornton et al., 2012). Thornton et al. (2012) noted that low confidence in shopping ability was the strongest deterrent in healthy shopping. Many caregivers believe that they are too busy to be healthful after perceiving the additional effort and time needed to prepare healthful meals as compared to 'ready-made' meals (Hollywood et al., 2013) or fast-food. As compared with noncaregivers, caregivers had greater odds of engaging in negative health behaviors, such as regular soda and fast food consumption, placing them at a higher risk of morbidity (Hoffman, Lee, & Mendez-Luck, 2012), especially in the presence of caregiver burden (Silver, 2004). Burden is the stress that caregivers attribute to their caregiving responsibilities (Zarit, Reever, & Bach-Peterson, 1980). Caregiver burden generally places caregivers at an increased risk of morbidity and mortality (Ross et al., 2013), however caregivers may also turn to negative behaviors (e.g., smoking, drinking alcohol, etc.) to alleviate this burden (Silver, 2004), further increasing their risk of morbidity and mortality. Numerous studies (Blum & Sherman, 2010; Haley, 2003; Hoffman et al., 2012) have noted that providing care for someone has been linked to negative physical and psychological outcomes (e.g., immune suppression, depression, and anxiety). Depression and anger have been linked to physical health issues, as well as decreased well-being (Ali & Bokharey, 2015). Rullier et al. (2014) found that caregivers who reported depressive symptoms were more likely to present a poor nutritional status.

It is important to note that supply and demand of fast food has increased in the recent decades with environments containing more opportunities to obtain fast food (Thornton et al., 2012) and less prioritization of family meals (Watkinson-Powell et al., 2014). Greater convenience of fast food (Thornton et al., 2012) and lack of healthy stores or healthy options in supermarkets may influence healthy behaviors. Caregivers reported purchasing unhealthy foods through impulse or habitual buying, as well as social pressure to decide upon an item without spending too long reading food labels (Hollywood et al., 2013). Furthermore, caregivers must consider food preferences of the entire family; making it difficult to make healthful meals that satisfy everyone (Watkinson-Powell et al., 2014). Finding dishes that the entire family would eat reinforces the tendency to stick to a core of select dishes (Stead et al., 2004), despite the need to consume a wide variety of foods to ensure a balance of nutrients (ADA, 2000). An individual's determination can spark motivation to eat healthier, but family and social contacts can influence his/her motivation to continue to eat healthier (Thornton et al., 2012). Barre et al. (2011) found that a lack of social support, or individuals to discuss healthy eating, was a barrier for pursuing healthy eating behaviors. Acknowledging the numerous barriers to healthy eating, one must recognize that dealing with any one barrier to nutrition or dietary change is unlikely to radically alter future dietary behavior or influence structural barriers to healthy eating (Stead et al., 2004).

3.2 Age Associated Dietary Changes

Although older adults' nutritional needs are about the same as younger adults, some changes do occur as individuals age. Understanding older adults' nutrition needs and guidelines for meeting these needs can help caregivers plan meals which can increase older care recipients' resilience.

3.2.1 Calories

Calorie needs decrease with age due to declines in muscle mass (which has a higher metabolic rate than body fat), and a tendency for physical activity to decrease with age. Meal planning is important to ensure older adults get the nutrients they need in fewer calories (Academy of Nutrition and Dietetics [AND], 2012). Consuming too many calories can result in weight gain. Excess weight is associated with many health concerns such as heart disease, high blood pressure and diabetes. Watching portion sizes and limiting intake of foods high in saturated fat and added sugar can help with weight control (Whitney & Rolfes, 2013). However, many older adults do not eat enough food, especially nutrient dense foods. As a result, they may not get enough calories or nutrients to maintain health. Unintentional weight loss is a major health concern for older adults (Gaddey & Holder, 2014).

3.2.2 Carbohydrate

The main function of carbohydrate in the body is to provide energy. Adequate carbohydrate is needed so protein will not be used for energy. Recommended carbohydrate intake is 45–65% of calories. Most carbohydrate should come from nutrient dense carbohydrate foods such as whole grains, vegetables, fruits, and legumes. Recommendations are to limit foods high in added sugar (Whitney & Rolfes, 2013).

3.2.3 Fiber

Dietary fiber is helpful for many conditions such as constipation, diarrhea, diverticulitis, heart disease, colon cancer, and diabetes. Food sources of fiber include whole grains, vegetables, fruits and legumes. Recommendations are that at least half of grains consumed should be whole grains (U.S. Department of Health and Human Services and U.S. Department of Agriculture (USDHHS & USDA, 2015)). For adults, the Dietary Reference Intake (DRI) for fiber is 14 g of fiber per 1000 calories (Whitney & Rolfes, 2013). Dietary fiber intake should be increased slowly. Increasing dietary fiber too fast can cause gas and pain. Fiber absorbs water; thus, it is important to consume adequate fluids when increasing fiber in the diet. Before increasing dietary fiber, older adults should check with their health care provider, especially if they have chewing, swallowing, stomach or intestinal problems (Whitney & Rolfes, 2013).

3.2.4 Protein

Protein has many functions in the body. Protein is needed for maintaining and repairing body tissues, wound healing, making enzymes and hormones, sustaining the immune system, fighting infections, and prevent muscle wasting. In fact, protein needs may increase with illness or surgery (Whitney & Rolfes, 2013). For adults, the DRI for protein is 0.8 g/kg body weight. However, research shows older adults may need more protein (1.0–1.5 g/kg). Because calorie needs decrease with age, recommendations are to consume lean, high-quality protein such as fish, poultry, lean meats, eggs, and low-fat dairy. Unfortunately, many older adults limit protein foods due to problems chewing or swallowing, cost, or difficulties with food preparation. However, protein foods are an important part of a healthful diet (Bernstein & Munoz, 2016).

3.2.5 Fat

Fats also have many roles in the body. Fats provide a concentrated source of energy, help to make cell membranes, provide essential fatty acids the body cannot make, and transport fat-soluble vitamins. Although fats are important, many people consume too much fat in their diet. High fat diets are linked to heart disease and obesity which can indirectly increase risk of diabetes and high blood pressure (Whitney & Rolfes, 2013). Recommendations are to consume less than 10% of calories from saturated fat, keep *trans*-fat as low as possible, and keep total fat intake between 20 and 35% of calories. It is also recommended that most fats should come from unsaturated fats (USDHHS & USDA, 2015). Fat intake can be decreased by choosing lean protein foods and low-fat dairy, using low-fat food preparation methods, and watching portion sizes of foods higher in fat (Bernstein & Munoz, 2016).

3.2.6 Vitamins and Minerals

Older adults have about the same vitamin and mineral needs as younger adults. However, some changes do occur with age. Sodium needs decrease with age and for women after menopause, iron needs decrease. Calcium, vitamin D, and vitamin B6 needs increase (Whitney & Rolfes, 2013). Stomach acid tends to decrease with age. In addition, atrophic gastritis is a condition that tends to occur with age. As a result, many older adults lose the ability to absorb naturally occurring vitamin B12 from food. Vitamin B12 deficiency can result in cognitive decline and irreversible nerve damage. Older adults are better able to absorb vitamin B12 from fortified foods or dietary supplements (Bernstein & Munoz, 2016). In addition to some changes in nutrient needs with age, older adults tend to have low dietary intakes of some nutrients including calcium, vitamin D, vitamin B12, vitamin E, potassium, zinc and fiber (AND, 2012; Bernstein & Munoz, 2016). Following a healthy dietary pattern is important to getting all the nutrients needed in the appropriate calorie level.

3.2.7 Water

Recommended fluid intake for adults and older adults is 1.0–1.5 mL/calorie with a minimum of 1500 mg (6 cups) daily. Additional fluid is needed to replace losses due to illness and extreme heat or humidity. Water can come in many forms such as water, juice, milk, etc. Although caffeine has a diuretic effect, in moderation, caffeinated beverages can count towards fluid intake. Alcohol results in extreme fluid loss and should not be counted towards fluid intake (Whitney & Rolfes, 2013).

3.3 Age-Associated Changes in Food Intake

As previously mentioned, understanding older adults' nutrition needs and guidelines for meeting those needs can help caregivers plan meals which can promote the care recipient's well-being; increasing their resilience. Caregivers should notify the older care recipients' health care provider if they do not feel the care recipient is able to consume a healthful diet.

3.3.1 Appetite

Decreased appetite is a common problem for many older adults, hindering their ability to obtain good nutrition, resulting in unexplained muscle loss, weight loss, dehydration, and malnutrition. Numerous factors (i.e., physical and socioemotional changes, medication use) can impact appetite (AND, 2012). Age-associated changes in taste and smell may decrease food appeal resulting in lower nutrient intake (ADA, 2000; Wellman, 2004). Changes in appetite regulation, such as low prioritization of meal times (Watkinson-Powell et al., 2014), can result in decreased hunger and early and prolonged feelings of fullness, resulting in decreased food intake (Donini, Savina, & Cannella, 2003). Maintaining the enjoyment of food, in addition to the social aspects, helps to minimize the risk of weight loss and contributes to quality of life (ADA, 2000). Loneliness in older adults can decrease one's motivation to prepare and eat healthy meals (Donini et al., 2003). Loneliness is not just related to living alone. Someone who lives with others, but does not have frequent communication may be lonelier than someone who lives alone, but has frequent communication (Klinenberg, 2016). Depression is also a common problem with aging. Depression is often overlooked among older adults because some of the signs of depression such as tiredness, irritability, confusion, or attention problems are viewed as aspects of aging (Gitlin, Chernett, Dennis, & Hauck, 2012). Depression often results from loneliness associated with the loss of family or friends (ADA, 2000), a sense of purpose, and use of certain medications. Health and financial problems can also contribute to depression (AND, 2012; de Castro, 2002). Diet and depression are interrelated. Depression can be caused by many nutrient deficiencies, such as vitamin B12 and folate (Tiemeier et al., 2002), which can lead to a decreased interest in preparing and eating food leading to a poorer diet. This can begin a downward spiral of further depression, poorer diet, and increased nutrient deficiency (Bailly, Maitre, & Van Wymelbeke, 2015), as well as an increased risk of limiting functional ability (ADA, 2000; Amarantos et al., 2001).

Older adults are more likely to take many medications for extended periods than other age groups (Kantor, Rehm, & Haas, 2015). Medications can affect taste as well as cause nausea, decreased appetite, and depressive symptoms, all of which decrease overall food intake (AND, 2012; Wellman, 2004). The American Dietetics Association (2000) cites polypharmacy as one of the most frequent nutritional risk factors in older adults. Nutritional concerns should be discussed with physicians, especially when discussing medication side effects. Eating a healthful diet can provide all the nutrients needed for health and well-being. Regular social interactions and regular physical activity can also provide emotional benefits and help to prevent illness and mobility problems which can further contribute to depression (Hertzog, Kramer, Wilson, & Lindenberger, 2008).

3.3.2 Thirst

Dehydration is a common and serious problem for many older adults. The thirst sensation tends to decrease with age, resulting in a decreased awareness of thirst, putting older adults at risk for dehydration (Juan & Basiotis, 2004). Other factors putting older adults at higher risk for dehydration include age-related decrease in muscle mass, body water and kidney function as well as self-limiting fluid intake due to swallowing problems, fear of incontinence, or decreased mobility (Hooper, Bunn, Jimoh, & Fairweather-Tait, 2014). Many symptoms of dehydration are misinterpreted as common signs of aging such as weakness, dry mouth, constipation, headache, irritability, sleepiness, and confusion (Wellman, 2004). Dehydration can also increase risk of urinary tract infections, pressure sores, and pneumonia.

3.3.3 Chewing and Swallowing

Several oral problems tend to increase with age. Common diet related oral problems include dry mouth, tooth decay, periodontal disease, and tooth loss (Bernstein & Munoz, 2016). Saliva tends to decrease with age. Saliva moistens food and makes swallowing easier. Decreased saliva and certain medications can result in dry mouth making it hard to taste, chew, and swallow (Turner & Ship, 2007). Poor dental hygiene is the main cause of tooth decay; however, diet can have an indirect role in tooth decay. Carbohydrate foods that tend to stick to the teeth can particularly promote decay. In addition, frequently eating and drinking sugary foods and beverages provides a constant source of food for bacteria. Limiting intake of sugary beverages and foods, especially between meals, can help reduce tooth decay (American Dietetic Association [ADA], 2007). Periodontal disease can damage the bone and tissues that support the teeth which can lead to tooth loss. Although bacterial infection is the cause of gum disease, many health conditions including diabetes, poor nutrition, and a weakened immune system can increase the rate and severity of the disease. Overall good nutrition is needed to support the body's immune system, fight infections, and help wounds heal (ADA, 2007; Scrimshaw & SanGiovanni, 1997). Tooth decay and periodontal disease can lead to tooth loss which can make chewing difficult increasing risk of choking. Many older adults are unable to adjust to dentures or have dentures that do not fit. In addition, dentures are not as effective for chewing as natural teeth (ADA, 2007). As a result, people who have lost teeth often choose foods that are soft and easy to chew. This can lead to increased intake of refined carbohydrates (which tend to be higher in fat, added sugar and calories) and decreased intake of fresh vegetables, fruits, whole grains, and protein foods. Over time limited food choices can lead to a poor quality diet (Walls & Steele, 2004). Difficulty swallowing is also a common problem for many older adults. In addition to decreased saliva and tooth loss, swallowing difficulty can be a consequence of stroke or other neurological problems. Age-related physical changes in tongue and throat strength and throat dilation can result in swallowing difficulties (Lancaster, 2015).

3.3.4 Energy, Strength, Coordination, and Range of Motion

Muscle mass tends to decrease with age. Muscle loss can result in decreased strength lowering one's ability to grocery shop, cook and eat. Combined muscle loss and decreased strength can affect ones' ability to move and maintain balance which can increase risk of falls (Bernstein & Munoz, 2016). Some estimates are that one-third of older adults' will fall each year which is a major cause of older adult injuries. Fear of falling may cause older adults to limit physical activity; however, decreased physical activity can actually result in decreased physical fitness further increasing risk of falls (Centers for Disease Control and Prevention, 2016). Regular physical activity, especially muscle-strengthening activity can help to preserve and build muscle (Denison, Cooper, Sayer, & Robinson, 2015). The Physical Activity Guidelines recommend older adults participate in at least 150 min of moderate-intensity physical activity a week and muscle-strengthening activities on 2 days a week. Recommendations for older adults who cannot meet these guidelines are to be as active as their abilities and conditions allow. Older adults are also encouraged to do activities to maintain or improve balance if they are at risk of falling (U.S. Department of Health and Human Services, 2008). Muscle also contains a large amount of water. In fact, up to 75% of muscle weight is water; therefore, muscle loss also results in a loss of body water placing older adults at increased risk of dehydration (Juan & Basiotis, 2004). Thus, by helping to maintain muscle, regular physical activity can also help to maintain body water. In addition to physical activity, older adults need adequate calories and protein to maintain muscle (Denison et al., 2015). Unfortunately, with age, calorie needs decline, primarily due to decreases in muscle mass and physical activity, while nutrient needs remain about the same. This emphasizes the importance of meal planning to ensure older adults get the nutrients they need in fewer calories (AND, 2012).

3.3.5 Bones and Joints

Bones are continually being broken down and rebuilt. In early life, up to about age 30, bones are built faster than they are broken down. However, in later life, after about age 30–40, bones are broken down faster than they are built. Although men and women both lose bone with age, women undergo a rapid rate of bone loss after menopause. In addition to normal decreases in bone formation with age, it is important to understand that the body requires calcium for many other body functions besides maintaining bones. If dietary calcium intake is adequate to meet the other body needs, excess calcium is deposited in the bones. However, if dietary calcium intake is not adequate to meet the other body needs, calcium is released from the bones which can further result in bone loss. Continual bone loss overtime can increase risk of osteoporosis, a condition where the bones become so thin and weak they easily fracture or break. The wrist, spine and hip are the most common bones to fracture. Bone fractures, especially of the hip and spine, can result in complications which unfortunately can decrease independence and quality of life (Whitney & Rolfes, 2013). Calcium and vitamin D are important for building and maintaining bones. However, many nutrients such as vitamin C, vitamin K, phosphorous, copper, zinc, magnesium and potassium are also needed to build and maintain healthy bones (Ilich, Brownbill, & Tamborini, 2003; Whitney & Rolfes, 2013). The role of so many nutrients for bone health further emphasizes the importance of consuming an overall healthful diet including a variety of foods. In addition to diet, regular physical activity, especially weight bearing physical activity, can help strengthen bones (Sochett, 2002). As previously mentioned, muscle-strengthening physical activities can help to maintain muscles and increase flexibility and balance which can help to prevent breaking bones due to falling (Bernstein & Munoz, 2016). Additional recommendations are to avoid smoking and excessive alcohol as these can increase bone loss (Sochett, 2002).

Arthritis (osteoarthritis and/or rheumatoid) is also a common joint problem with aging. Arthritis is inflammation of the joints which can result in pain, swelling, and even structural changes in the joints. These changes can have a tremendous impact on older adults' food intake by affecting their ability to grocery shop, cook, and even eat (Whitney & Rolfes, 2013). Experiences of arthritic pain from numerous trips to the toilet may contribute to older adults limiting fluid intake (Wellman, 2004).

3.3.6 Cognition

The range of 'normal cognitive aging' (Deary et al., 2009, p. 138) allows for some age-associated declines in cognition in some areas (e.g., memory, executive functions, processing speed, reasoning), while others remain relatively stable (e.g., numeric and language abilities, general knowledge). It is important to note most changes in cognitive function related to age are mild. In fact, memory loss is often due to depression rather than cognitive decline (Bernstein & Munoz, 2016). Nerve cells in the brain depend on many nutrients to function properly (Bourre, 2006). Confusion and memory loss may be due, in part, to nutrient deficiencies, such as vitamin B12, folate, and vitamin B6 (Barberger-Gateau, 2014; Mallidou & Cartie, 2015). As previously stated, vitamin B12 is already a nutrient of concern with aging due to atrophic gastritis. Dehydration can also result in confusion (Suhr, Hall, Patterson, & Niinisto, 2004).

Eating a healthful diet providing all the nutrients needed is important for helping to maintain cognitive function. In addition, both physical and mental activities that simulate the body and mind can help to maintain cognitive function (Rosenberg & Miller, 1992). In some cases, cognitive loss is extensive and grouped under the term dementia.

Dementia is a progressive condition characterized by impairment due to brain dysfunctioning in at least three spheres (i.e., memory, cognition, language, personality, visuospatial skills, emotions) (Ali & Bokharey, 2015). Vascular dementia is caused by atherosclerosis or micro-bleeds in the small blood vessels of the brain. Preventing or controlling atherosclerosis can help lower risk of vascular dementia (Bernstein & Munoz, 2016). Although Alzheimer's disease tends to have a genetic component; oxidative damage and high homocysteine levels may have a role in its development (Otaequi-Arrazola, Amiano, Elbusto, Urdaneta, & Martinez-Lage, 2013). Vegetables, fruits, whole grains and lean protein foods provide antioxidant nutrients which help reduce oxidative damage, as well as provide folate, vitamin B6, and vitamin B_{12} which can lower homocysteine (Whitney & Rolfes, 2013). The role of many nutrients in cognitive health, again, emphasized the importance of an overall healthful diet. Older adult cognitive decline is a major cause of weight loss. Decreased appetite, confusion, memory loss, and difficult feeding behaviors are all associated with weight loss. If an individual is not eating enough their health care provider may recommend supplemental nutrition (AND, 2012).

3.4 Nutrition Implications for Resilience

Lack of proper nutrition has been linked to declines in functional status (Amarantos et al., 2001), limiting the individual's ability to engage in physical activity, thus increasing their risk for morbidity and mortality. As mentioned previously, these functional limitations can increase an individual's dependency on others to provide assistance. Adequate nutrition is vital for individuals to maintain good health, independence, and quality of life (ADA, 2000; Hermann et al., 2012). Good nutrition improves health related quality of life through prevention of dietary deficiency diseases and mitigating malnutrition associated with other diseases (Amarantos et al., 2001). This results in improved overall health, decreased dependency, reduced number of hospitalizations, reduced recuperation time and a reduction in health care resource utilization; benefiting both the individual and society (ADA, 2000). It is important to note that caregivers can have a direct impact on their care recipients' well-being.

Caregivers assist their care recipients with purchasing groceries and preparing meals, thus they have the ability to influence healthy choices. An important determinant in healthy food choices was the caregiver's self-perception of his/her cooking skills (Stead et al., 2004; Watkinson-Powell et al., 2014). Caregivers who expressed confidence in their cooking skills were more willing to attempt preparing a wide variety of dishes than those who expressed no confidence. The caregiver's ability to prepare healthy choices can either offer protection or be a vulnerability for the care recipient. As mentioned previously, a wide variety of dishes allows for greater intake of nutrients which in turn promotes health. However, caregivers with low cooking skills may rely heavily on fast food or frozen and pre-prepared foods (Stead et al., 2004) that are low in micronutrients (Thornton et al., 2012). This lack of food choices, in conjunction with low prioritization of mealtimes, can compromise nutritional care (Watkinson-Powell et al., 2014). Eating is not just a biological role, but one that also contains social and emotional components (Rullier et al., 2013), providing both sensory and psychological pleasures (Amarantos et al., 2001). Thornton et al. (2012) state that members of a household can influence the motivation of other family members to eat healthy, as well as provide healthy options by modeling this behavior at regular family meals. Locher, Robinson, Roth, Ritchie, and Burgio (2005) studied the influence of individuals' presence during meals on the caloric intake of older adults. Their results showed that when an individual was present during the meal, the older adult consumed an average of 114 more calories per meal than when an individual was not present. The authors speculated that the presence of another individual may extend the length of the meal, allowing the individual more time to eat. It is also likely that the individual may have offered encouragement to the care recipient to continue eating.

Cases of dementia may increase the caregiving dyads' vulnerability. Due to the interindividual variability in dementia patients resulting from impairment in various brain regions (Ali & Bokharey, 2015), it is difficult to pinpoint the exact symptomology that care recipients may experience. Caregivers often have limited knowledge about dementia symptoms and may incorrectly interpret symptoms as difficult behaviors, especially during mealtimes (Rullier et al., 2014). Ali and Bokharey (2015) note that the dyad's quality of life, and resultant resilience, is dependent upon the caregivers' ability to adapt to needs and behaviors of the care recipient. Thus caregivers who are slow to adapt to their care recipient's behaviors may negatively affect mealtime interactions, weakening the psychosocial function of eating with other persons (Rullier et al., 2014). Due to intellectual impairment, individuals with dementia have difficulty understanding and expressing their own needs and wants (Rullier et al., 2013), thus many caregivers make decisions for them, such as food choices. This lack of choice slowly begins to remove the older adult's sense of empowerment. Johnston, Brosi, Hermann, and Jaco (2011) described empowerment as countless experiences that promote feelings of power, authority, and self-worth, leading to a sense of perceived control. Providing choices for the older adult can help in nutrition (Watkinson-Powell et al., 2014), as well as increasing the care recipient's quality of life, thwarting the risk of an older adult internalizing beliefs of little self-worth and creating a poor self-conception (Johnston et al., 2011).

3.5 Tools and Resources

3.5.1 2015–2020 Dietary Guidelines for Americans

The 2015–2020 Dietary Guidelines can help individuals make food choices to have a healthier diet. Healthful eating not only promotes health, but also helps to decrease risk of chronic disease. The Dietary Guidelines recommend consuming a healthful diet at an appropriate calorie level. A healthful diet includes a variety of vegetables, fruits, grains, fat-free or low-fat dairy, and a variety of protein foods and oils. A healthful diet also includes limited amounts of saturated fats and *trans* fats, added sugars, and sodium (USDHHS & USDA, 2015).

3.5.2 MyPlate Daily Checklist

MyPlate is the U.S. Department of Agriculture's food group symbol. The MyPlate symbol is a reminder to make healthy food choices (USDA, 2016). The MyPlate Daily Checklist is a guide to plan a healthful diet and is based on the 2015–2020 Dietary Guidelines for Americas. The MyPlate Daily Checklist provides recommendations for the amount of food from each MyPlate food group and limits for fats, added sugars and sodium based on estimated calorie needs. Personalized eating patterns at 12 calorie levels can be found at http://www.choosemyplate.gov/MyPlate-Daily-Checklist-input (USDA, n.d.).

3.5.3 Dietary Supplements

Older adults can get the nutrients they need by eating a variety of foods following the MyPlate Daily Checklist. The more variety, the less likely one is to get too much or too little of a nutrient. However, many physical factors as well as social and emotional changes and limited finances can cause older adults to eat less or have a poor diet. Older adults with these issues may benefit from a dietary supplement (AND, 2012). When choosing a dietary supplement, caregivers should look for one with a variety of vitamins and minerals and no more than 100% of recommended amounts. Do not take vitamins or minerals in large amounts unless advised by a health care provider. It is easier to get too much of a vitamin or mineral from a supplement than from food, and too much of a nutrient can cause problems (Food and Drug Administration [FDA], 2002). It's important to realize that not all claims on dietary supplements are FDA approved (Food and Drug Administration [FDA], 2016a). Unlike drugs, dietary supplements are not tested for safety before they are allowed to be sold. It is also important to realize that dietary supplements do not make up for a poor diet as they do not provide the calories, carbohydrate, protein, fats, fiber and other compounds important for health (Food and Drug Administration [FDA], 2016b).

> **Breakout Box 3.1 Focus on Practice**
> The process of aging brings with it rewards and challenges that require new information to improve our understanding of dealing with the changing seasons of our lives. Perhaps nowhere is the value of useful information more relevant than caregiving for an older adult family member or older adults in general. The older person's mind may hold on to memories of the ways and what that they ate in bygone days and these memories may outweigh their current physical or nutritional needs and challenges. To address these challenges and finding new ways of assisting older persons in changing eating behaviors, a dietitian and behavioral aide from a continuing care retirement center offered advice on older adult feeding practices. Routines are important among older adults such as consistent meal times, portion sizes, eating with the same people at the same table, and providing community oriented information during meals. These steps taken at home while older adults remain independent will assist in future transitions to continuing care. The appropriateness of the older adult's plate and its contents must be reviewed consistently as inevitable physiological challenges may require the introduction of new foods, attention to nutritional needs, consumption facilitating preparation techniques, portion sizes, and support in feeding aligned. All of these changes are best supported by developing strong routines. Likewise, emphasize the importance of caregivers stepping back frequently and observing how well an older adult is eating and address any difficulties. Make sure that some of those favorite old foods from the past have their place on the plate from time to time, even if modified for easier chewing and swallowing. Share memories, develop routines by developing mealtime rituals and traditions will assist caregivers in ensuring that meal time is a favorite time for older adults. Planned mealtime will also help to ensure a longer life for older adults and more gratification with the outcomes of caregiving for family members and professionals.
> —From notes taken during conversations with food service personnel working at various levels at four assisted living facilities.

3.5.4 Ten Tips for Healthy Nutrition

Ten tips have been provided to help promote healthy nutrition and social interactions between members of the caregiving dyad.

1. Have meals at regular times and provide ample time for meal consumption.
2. Serve a variety at meals.
3. Invite family and friends over for meals.
4. Encourage physical activity to increase appetite and maintain strength.
5. Be aware of medication side effects.

6. Encourage safety in the kitchen and allow your loved one to assist.
7. Have plenty of fluids available at meals and throughout the day to promote hydration.
8. Keep a supply of healthy foods on hand for days you do not feel like shopping.
9. If feeding an individual, remember to feed small amounts of food and allow ample time for chewing. Be sure to preserve your loved one's dignity!
10. Talk with your doctor if you believe your loved one is not getting the nutrition they need.

3.6 Conclusions and Future Directions

Good nutrition has an important role in maintaining older adults' quality of life. Healthy lifestyle behaviors, including good nutrition, can help promote health and lower risk of some age-related conditions. It is important to acknowledge that individuals must be motivated to make healthy choices. Many individuals note that dietary guidelines are not specifically disseminated for consumers to implement while shopping (Hollywood et al., 2013). Caregivers need adequate information and training in order to provide older care recipients' appropriate nutritional support. Caregivers may benefit from training on how to provide proper nutrition support for various health conditions, modify foods, supplemental nutrition, and techniques and coping skills when feeding others. Information on the importance of the caregiver's own health and emotional well-being, as well as available resources, are also extremely important (AND, 2012).

Questions for Thought and Discussion
1. What older adult body systems does diet affect?
2. What older adult body systems does physical activity affect?
3. How are body systems interrelated with health conditions, such as with dehydration and food borne illness?
4. Why are older adults' overall diet emphasized over individual nutrients?

Glossary

Dietary Reference Intake (DRI)	The Dietary Reference Intakes are estimates of the amount of nutrients needed by healthy people.
Essential fatty acids	Essential fatty acids are fatty acids the body cannot make and therefore they must come from the diet.
Inflammation	Inflammation is a localized reaction to an injury or infection.
MyPlate Daily Checklist	The MyPlate Daily Checklist is a guide to the amount of foods to consume from each MyPlate food group based on calorie level.

MyPlate food groups	The MyPlate food groups are grains, vegetables, fruit, dairy, and protein foods.
Oxidative damage	Oxidative damage is tissue damage caused by free radicals.
Saturated fats	Saturated fats are a type of fatty acid that do not contain double bonds.
Trans fats	*Trans* fats are a type of unsaturated fatty acids often produced during the process of hydrogenation.

References

Academy of Nutrition and Dietetics. (2012). Position of the Academy of Nutrition and Dietetics: Food and nutrition for older adults: Promoting health and wellness. *Journal of the Academy of Nutrition and Dietetics, 112*, 1255–1277. doi:10.1016/j.jand.2012.06.015

Acton, G. J. (2002). Health-promoting self-care in family caregivers. *Western Journal of Nursing Research, 24*, 73–86. doi:10.1177/01939450222045716

Ali, S., & Bokharey, I. Z. (2015). Efficacy of cognitive behavior therapy among caregivers of dementia: An outcome study. *Pakistan Journal of Psychological Research, 30*, 249–269. Retrieved from http://www.pjprnip.edu.pk/pjpr/index.php/pjpr/article/download/340/351

Amarantos, E., Martinez, A., & Dwyer, J. (2001). Nutrition and quality of life in older adults. *Journals of Gerontology: Series A, 56A*, 54–64. Retrieved from https://www.ncbi.nlm.nih.gov/pubmed/11730238

American Dietetic Association. (2000). Position of the American Dietetic Association: Nutrition, aging, and the continuum of care. *Journal of the American Dietetic Association, 100*, 580–595. doi:10.1016/S0002-8223(00)00177-2

American Dietetic Association. (2007). Position of the American Dietetic Association: Oral health and nutrition. *Journal of the American Dietetic Association, 107*, 1418–1428. doi:10.1016/j.jada.2007.06.003

Bailly, N., Maitre, I., & Van Wymelbeke, V. (2015). Relationships between nutritional status, depression and pleasure of eating in aging men and women. *Archives of Gerontology and Geriatrics, 61*, 330–336. doi:10.1016/j.archger.2015.08.020

Barberger-Gateau, P. (2014). Nutrition and brain aging: How can we move ahead? *European Journal of Clinical Nutrition, 68*, 1245–1249. doi:10.1038/ejcn.2014.177

Barre, L. K., Ferron, J. C., Davis, K. E., & Whitley, R. (2011). Healthy eating in persons with serious mental illnesses: Understanding and barriers. *Psychiatric Rehabilitation Journal, 34*, 304–310. doi:10.2975/34.4.2011.304.310

Bernstein, M., & Munoz, N. (2016). *Nutrition for the older adult*. Burlington: Jones & Partlett Learning.

Blum, K., & Sherman, D. W. (2010). Understanding the experience of caregivers: A focus on transitions. *Seminars in Oncology Nursing, 26*, 243–258. doi:10.1016/j.soncn.2010.08.005

Bourre, J. M. (2006). Effects of nutrients (in food) on the structure and function of the nervous system: Update on dietary requirements for the brain. *Journal of Nutrition, Health and Aging, 10*, 377–385. Retrieved from http://www.bourre.fr/pdf/publications_scientifiques/259.pdf

Castro, C. M., King, A. C., Housemann, R., Bacak, S. J., McMullen, K. M., & Brownson, R. C. (2007). Rural family caregivers and health behaviors: Results from an epidemiologic survey. *Journal of Aging and Health, 19*, 87–105. doi:10.1177/0898264306296870

Centers for Disease Control and Prevention. (2016, January 20). *Important facts about falls*. Retrieved from http://www.cdc.gov/HomeandRecreationalSafety/Falls/adultfalls.html

de Castro, J. M. (2002). Age-related changes in the social, psychological, and temporal influences on food intake in free-living healthy, adult humans. *Journal of Gerontology, 57A*, M368–M377. doi:10.1093/gerona/57.6.M368

Deary, I. J., Corley, J., Gow, A. J., Harris, S. E., Houlihan, L. M., Marioni, R. E., ... Starr, J. M. (2009). Age-associated cognitive decline. *British Medical Bulletin, 92*, 135–152. doi:10.1093/bmb/ldp033

Denison, H. J., Cooper, C., Sayer, A. A., & Robinson, S. M. (2015). Prevention and optimal management of sarcopenia: A review of combined exercise and nutrition interventions to improve muscle outcomes in older people. *Clinical Interventions in Aging, 10*, 859–869. doi:10.2147/CIA.S55842

Donini, L. M., Savina, C., & Cannella, C. (2003). Eating habits and appetite control in the elderly: The anorexia of aging. *International Psychogeriatrics, 15*, 973–987. doi:10.1017/S1041610203008779

Food and Drug Administration. (2002, January). *Tips for dietary supplement users*. Retrieved from http://www.fda.gov/Food/DietarySupplements/UsingDietarySupplements/ucm110567.htm

Food and Drug Administration. (2016a, April 11). *Label claims for conventional foods and dietary supplements*. Retrieved from http://www.fda.gov/food/ingredientspackaginglabeling/labelingnutrition/ucm111447.htm

Food and Drug Administration. (2016b, January 13). *Information for consumers on using dietary supplements*. Retrieved from http://www.fda.gov/Food/DietarySupplements/UsingDietarySupplements/default.htm

Gaddey, H. L., & Holder, K. (2014). Unintentional weight loss in older adults. *American Family Physician, 80*, 718–722.

Gitlin, L. N., Chernett, N. L., Dennis, M. P., & Hauck, W. W. (2012). Identification if and beliefs about depressive symptoms and preferred treatment approaches among community-living older African Americans. *American Journal of Geriatric Psychiatry, 20*, 973–984. doi:10.1097/JGP.0b013e31825463ce

Haley, W. E. (2003). The costs of family caregiving: Implications for geriatric oncology. *Critical Reviews in Oncology and Hematology, 48*, 151–158. doi:10.1016/j.critrevonc.2003.04.005

Hermann, J. R., Brosi, W. A., Johnston, J. H., & Jaco, L. (2012). Formative assessment of assistance needed with grocery shopping and preparing food among rural community-dwelling older adults. *Journal of Extension, 50*, 1–8. Retrieved from https://www.joe.org/joe/2012february/rb5.php

Hertzog, C., Kramer, A. F., Wilson, R. S., & Lindenberger, U. (2008). Enrichment effects on adult cognitive development: Can the functional capacity of older adults be preserved and enhanced? *Psychological Science in the Public Interest, 9*, 1–65. doi:10.1111/j.1539-6053.2009.01034.x

Hoffman, G. J., Lee, J., & Mendez-Luck, C. A. (2012). Health behaviors among Baby Boomer informal caregivers. *The Gerontologist, 52*, 219–230. doi:10.1093/geront/gns003

Hollywood, L. E., Cuskelly, G. J., O'Brien, M., McConnon, A., Barnett, J., Raats, M. M., & Dean, M. (2013). Healthful grocery shopping. Perceptions and barriers. *Appetite, 70*, 119–126. doi:10.1016/j.appet.2013.03.090

Hooper, L., Bunn, D., Jimoh, F. O., & Fairweather-Tait, S. J. (2014). Water-loss dehydration and aging. *Mechanisms of Ageing and Development, 136–137*, 50–58. doi:10.1016/j.mad.2013.11.09

Ilich, J., Brownbill, R., & Tamborini, L. (2003). Bone and nutrition in elderly women: Protein, energy, and calcium as main determinants of bone mineral density. *European Journal of Clinical Nutrition, 57*, 554–565. doi:10.1038/sj.ejcn.1601577

Johnston, J. H., Brosi, W. A., Hermann, J. R., & Jaco, L. (2011). The impact of social support on perceived control among older adults: Building blocks of empowerment. *Journal of Extension, 49*, 1–8. Retrieved from https://www.joe.org/joe/2011october/rb4.php

Juan, W., & Basiotis, P. (2004). More than one in three older Americans may not drink enough water. *Family Economics & Nutrition Review, 16*, 49–51.

Kantor, E. D., Rehm, C. D., & Haas, J. S. (2015). Trends in prescription drug use among adults in the United States from 1999-2012. *Journal of the American Medical Association, 314*, 1818–1830. doi:10.1001/jama.2015.13766

Kendall, P. A., Hillers, V. V., & Medeiros, L. C. (2006). Food safety guidance for older adults. *Clinical Infectious Diseases, 42*, 1298–1304. doi:10.1086/503262

Klinenberg, E. (2016). Social isolation, loneliness, and living alone: Identifying the risks for public health. *American Journal of Public Health, 106*, 786–787. doi:10.2105/AHPH.2016.303166

Lancaster, J. (2015). Dysphagia: Its nature, assessment and management. *British Journal of Community Nursing, 20*, S28–S32. doi:10.12968/bjcn.2015.20.Sup6a.S28

Locher, J. L., Robinson, C. O., Roth, D. L., Ritchie, C. S., & Burgio, K. L. (2005). The effect of the presence of others on caloric intake in homebound older adults. *Journal of Gerontology: Medical Sciences, 60A*, 1475–1478. doi:10.1093/Gerona/60.11.1475

Mallidou, A., & Cartie, M. (2015). Nutritional habits and cognitive performance of older adults. *Nursing Management, 22*, 27–43. doi:10.7748/nm.22.3.27.e1331

National Alliance on Caregiving, & AARP Public Policy Institute. (2015). *Caregiving in the U.S. 2015*. Retrieved from http://www.caregiving.org/caregiving2015/

Otaequi-Arrazola, A., Amiano, P., Elbusto, A., Urdaneta, E., & Martinez-Lage, P. (2013). Diet, cognition, and Alzheimer's disease: Food for thought. *European Journal of Nutrition, 53*, 1–23. doi:10.1007/s00394-013-0561-3

Rosenberg, I. H., & Miller, J. W. (1992). Nutritional factors in physical and cognitive functions of elderly people. *American Journal of Clinical Nutrition, 55*, 1237S–1243S.

Ross, A., Sundaramurthi, T., & Bevans, M. (2013). A labor of love: The influence of cancer caregiving on health behaviors. *Cancer Nursing, 36*, 474–483. doi:10.1097/NCC.0b013e3182747b75

Rullier, L., Lagarde, A., Bouisson, J., Bergua, V., & Barberger-Gateau, P. (2013). Nutritional status of community-dwelling older people with dementia: Associations with individual and family caregivers' characteristics. *International Journal of Geriatric Psychiatry, 28*, 580–588. doi:10.1002/gps.3862

Rullier, L., Lagarde, A., Bouisson, J., Bergua, V., Torres, M., & Barberger-Gateau, P. (2014). Psychosocial correlates of nutritional status of family caregivers of persons with dementia. *International Psychogeriatrics, 26*, 105–113. doi:10.1017/S1041610213001579

Scrimshaw, N. S., & SanGiovanni, J. P. (1997). Synergism of nutrition, infection, and immunity: An overview. *American Journal of Clinical Nutrition, 66*, 464S–477S.

Silver, H. J. (2004). The nutrition-related needs of family caregivers. *Generations, 28*, 61–64. Retrieved from http://search.proquest.com/docview/212223381?accountid=4117

Silver, H. J., & Wellman, N. S. (2002). Nutrition education may reduce burden in family caregivers of older adults. *Journal of Nutrition Education and Behavior, 34*, S53–S58. doi:10.1016/s1499-4046(06)60312-6

Sochett, E. (2002). Healthy bones—Activity and nutrition. *Paediatrics & Child Health, 7*, 315–317.

Stead, M., Caraher, M., & Anderson, A. (2004). Confident, fearful, and hopeless cooks: Findings from the development of a food-skills initiative. *British Food Journal, 106*, 274–287. doi:10.1108/00070700410529546

Suhr, J.A., Hall, J., Patterson, S. M. & Niinisto, R. T. (2004). The relation of hydration status to cognitive performance in healthy older adults. *International Journal of Psychophysiology, 53*, 121–125. doi:10.1016/j.ijpsycho.2004.03.003

Thornton, L. E., Jeffery, R. W., & Crawford, D. A. (2012). Barriers to avoiding fast-food consumption in an environment supportive of unhealthy eating. *Public Health Nutrition, 16*, 2105–2113. doi:10.1017/S1368980012005083

Tiemeier, H., Ruud van Tuiji, H., Hofman, A., Meijer, J., Kiliaan, A. J., & Breteler, M. B. (2002). Vitamin B12, folate, and homocysteine in depression: The Rotterdam study. *American Journal of Psychiatry, 159*, 2099–2102. doi:10.1176/appi.ajp.159.12.2099

Turner, M. D., & Ship, J. A. (2007). Dry mouth and its effects on the oral health of elderly people. *The Journal of the American Dental Association, 138*, S15–S20. doi:10.14219/jada.archive.2007.0358

U.S. Department of Agriculture. (2016, January 7). *MyPlate*. Retrieved from http://www.choosemyplate.gov/MyPlate

U.S. Department of Agriculture. (n.d.). *MyPlate checklist calculator*. Retrieved from http://www.choosemyplate.gov/MyPlate-Daily-Checklist-input

U.S. Department of Health and Human Services. (2008). *2008 Physical activity guidelines for Americans* (ODPHP Publication No. U0036). Retrieved from http://health.gov/paguidelines/guidelines/default.aspx

U.S. Department of Health and Human Services and U.S. Department of Agriculture. (2015). *2015–2020 Dietary guidelines for Americans* (8th ed). Retrieved from http://health.gov/dietaryguidelines/2015/guidelines/

Walls, A. W. G., & Steele, J. G. (2004). The relationship between oral health and nutrition in older adults. *Mechanisms of Ageing and Development, 125*(12), 853–857. doi:10.1016/j.mad.2004.07.011

Watkinson-Powell, A., Barnes, S., Lovatt, M., Wasielewska, A., & Drummond, B. (2014). Food provision for older people receiving home care from the perspective of home-care workers. *Health and Social Care in the Community, 22*, 553–560. doi:10.1111/hsc.12117

Wellman, N. S. (2004). Nutrition and older adults—Why you should care talking to families and caregivers. *Generations, 28*, 97–99. Retrieved from http://search.proquest.com/docview/61365049/CB7CD721203E4277PQ/1?accountid=4117

Whitney, E., & Rolfes, S. R. (2013). *Understanding nutrition*. Belmont: Wadsworth.

Zarit, S. H., Reever, K. E., & Bach-Peterson, J. (1980). Relatives of the impaired elderly: Correlates of feelings of burden. *The Gerontologist, 20*, 649–655. doi:10.1093/geront/20.6.649

Chapter 4
Caregiver Resilience: Improving Ergonomics for the Safety, Comfort, and Health of Caregivers

Aditya Jayadas and Mihyun Kang

Hospitals and nursing homes are not always welcoming; instead of making patients and caregivers feel comfortable and supporting their health and wellbeing, they produce stress and anxiety. To identify and address issues such as stress in patients and caregivers, there is very little collaboration between environmental designers, researchers, hospital staff, patients and family caregivers (Rashid & Zimring, 2008). Basic needs of especially the caregiver, including comfortable sitting and sleeping are often not met in hospitals. Caregivers often sit long hours while attempting to take care of their loved ones, while being restricted to sleep on uncomfortable furniture in order to be in close proximity to the patients for whom they care. Such limitations and inadequacies in available accommodations for caregivers are not only uncomfortable, they can also be unsafe. Prolonged sitting with immobility in the knee and hip joints, and compression of the popliteal vein at the edge of the chair results in reduced venous blood flow (Oyama, Ebine, Ando, & Noro, 2004). Also, inadequate sleep can result from uncomfortable furniture and is directly associated with elevated worry and stress. Adequate sleep is a basic necessity and is widely accepted that 6–8 h of sleep is essential to maintain good health and function well in everyday activities (Dahl & Lewin, 2002). Inadequate sleep often leads to a diminished ability to think and make decisions. While it is challenging to address the many factors that contribute to caregiver stress, design for sleep comfort can be readily addressed through design interventions.

Lack of good ergonomically designed furniture can negatively impact the health and wellbeing of caregivers and possibly increase the risk of a caregiver becoming a patient themselves. Standard furniture is often placed in hospitals without a clear understanding of caregiver needs. Thus there is a *critical need* to develop novel and innovative furniture designs from an ergonomic standpoint so that caregivers can sit

---

A. Jayadas, Ph.D. (✉) • M. Kang, Ph.D.
Department of Design Housing and Merchandising, Oklahoma State University,
431 Human Sciences, Stillwater, OK 74078, USA
e-mail: aditya.jayadas@okstate.edu; mihyun.kang@okstate.edu

and sleep better. Two novel ergonomically designed furniture designs, namely a Venous Chair design and a Sit2Sleep design are being proposed to better address the needs of caregivers for seated and sleep related activities. It is anticipated that the newly designed furniture innovations will have a positive impact on the health and wellbeing of caregivers.

4.1 Introduction

Caregivers spend a large portion of their time sitting and sleeping. Though several caregiving activities are carried out while standing and moving around, this chapter focuses on caregiver challenges and risks, and ergonomic design interventions as they relate to sitting and sleeping.

4.1.1 Background

In a study of evidenced-based design in hospitals, Trochelman, Albert, Spence, Murray, and Slifcak (2012) reported that dissatisfying features in the patient room included: patient room size and location, bathroom, window size and placement, color used on the walls, lighting systems and acoustic control, signage, clock placement, television control and furniture. These factors can negatively impact the health and wellbeing of patients and caregivers alike. For instance, inappropriately designed furniture can result in uneven pressure at the ischial tuberosity (in the buttocks area) and thus cause low back pain due to poor posture. O'Keeffe, Dankaerts, O'Sullivan, O'Sullivan, and O'Sullivan (2013) reported that sitting related low back pain was significantly higher in a standard chair when compared to a dynamic forward inclined chair. Chairs that are ergonomically designed with several options for adjustability are often more expensive, therefore, cost considerations should be taken into account. An effective design intervention could consider the cushion material used in chairs. ProBax is one such intervention that is a patented system of foam inserts located in the base cushion. The Venous Chair (from Charles Alan Inc.) that has the patented ProBax cushion which is being proposed as a design intervention not only helps improve posture but also helps improve venous blood flow (Charles Alan, 2015).

An innovation such as the Venous Chair is especially important given the number of family caregivers in the United States. It is estimated that 43.5 million Americans provide care for an individual over the age of 50 (as cited in Giovannetti & Wolff, 2010). If the 43.5 million caregivers in America sat in a chair for an average of 90 min in a day that would total 3.9 billion hours of seated time. If a majority of that time is not spent being comfortable in a chair, the caregiver could become the patient. The number of caregivers is expected to continue to grow as there will be more number of older individuals with each progressing year. The Center for

Disease Control (CDC) reports that by 2030, 20% of the population in the United States will be over 65 years of age (CDC, 2013). The more alarming statistic is that two out of three older individuals will have multiple chronic conditions and treatment of this population will account for 66% of the budget. With older individuals living into their 80s and 90s and visiting hospitals multiple times in a year, an increase in the number of caregivers needed to take care of these individuals is inevitable.

As more family caregivers take on the active role of caregiving, it is important that they are comfortable when they sit and take care of their loved ones. Helander and Zhang (1997) have carried out field studies on comfort and discomfort in seated activities and have stressed the importance of comfort while seated for health and wellbeing of individuals. There have been several studies (Castellucci, Arezes, & Viviani, 2010; Dianat, Karimi, Hashemi, & Bahrampour, 2013; Gouvali & Boudolos, 2006; Molenbroek, Kroon-Ramaekers, & Snijders, 2003) on furniture carried out in schools to accommodate the needs of children, however, there is minimal research on furniture design in hospital settings to address the needs of adult caregivers. Most furniture in hospital settings has been designed without empathically considering the caregivers physical and psychological needs, or the importance of their role in care. Empathic design involves "stepping into the lives of individuals to better design for them" (Niinimaki & Koskinen, 2011). Without a clear understanding of caregiver needs, standard furniture has been placed in hospitals and nursing homes.

One of the approaches to assess comfort of furniture used by caregivers is to carry out a usability test. In a study evaluating the usability of military control chairs, the headrest, seatback, seat pan, armrest and controller were all evaluated for satisfaction using a 7-point Likert scale questionnaire when compared to an office chair and a bus seat (Lee et al., 2015). Lack of comfort as depicted by the satisfaction scores could result in pain or fatigue, and thus negatively affect the health and wellbeing of individuals using the chair. Variability in anthropometric dimensions of individuals also affects the usability scores when there is lack of adjustability in furniture, and standard furniture is used, like those placed in hospitals.

In addition to the placement of standardized furniture, there is often limited space in hospitals and nursing homes to accommodate the diverse tasks that caregivers are involved in. The 2010 Facility Guideline Institute's *Guidelines for Design and Construction of Health Care Facilities* (FGI) recommends that patient/family-centered patient rooms should include 250 ft^2 of clear floor area, exclusive of toilet rooms, closets, lockers, wardrobes, alcoves, or vestibules (Maolne & Dellinger, 2011). With limited space, multiple pieces of furniture cannot be accommodated in the room so a more flexible design allowing for multiple uses is essential. The Sit2Sleep design can be used for sitting, storage (in the sides), as a side table and most importantly for sleeping when stretched out full and the cushions folded out.

Therefore, a novel Venous Chair (see Fig. 4.1) and a Sit2Sleep furniture designed are being proposed. Both of these furniture items are expected to significantly improve the health and wellbeing of caregivers as they sit and sleep.

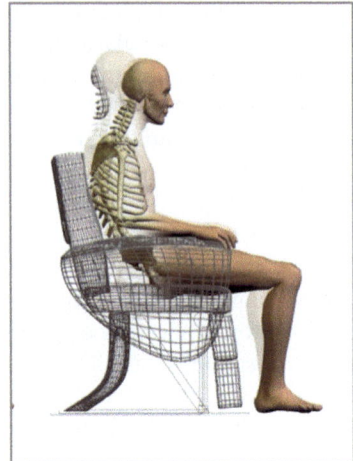 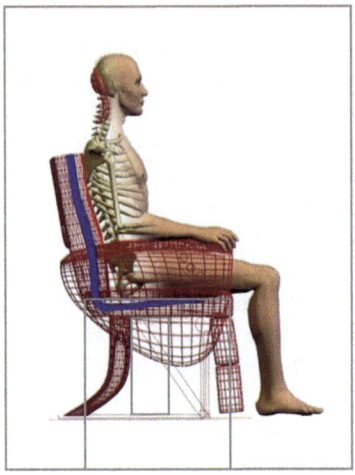

Conventional seat allowing the body to slump

Venous Chair with the ProBax seat holding the body in a more upright posture

Fig. 4.1 Conventional seating and Venous Chair with ProBax [Adapted from the ProBax brochure (with permission)]

4.1.2 Innovation

Venous stasis and long distance travel such as in airplanes has been explored in the past (Mittermayr et al., 2007; Oyama et al., 2004). However, there is a lack of understanding of venous blood flow during prolonged sitting of caregivers in hospital settings. It is expected that the novel Venous Chair design being proposed in the study will lead to improved venous blood flow as caregivers spend time seated beside their loved ones for whom they provide care. Such an intervention with a patented cushion will be especially useful for older individuals who have challenges with reduced blood flow. In terms of the specific design of the patented ProBax cushion (Patent # *US 20080079299 A1*) in the Venous Chair, a wedge shape design (refer Fig. 4.2) is what makes the cushion unique. The cushion is designed such that it starts off as thick toward the rear end (close to the seat pan near the back support) and it tapers toward the front of the seat. This improved posture resulting from sitting on the unique patented cushion embedded in the seat leads to reduced back pain, improved lung function, raised eye-line associated with improved social interaction and most importantly improved venous blood low (Charles Alan, 2015).

While sitting comfortably is of great importance for caregivers, the issue of sleep is of utmost importance as it relates to health and well-being. In a study of individuals caring for a person with dementia, Ding (2011) reported that sleep deficit was a good predictor of fatigue in caregivers, and negatively affected their health. A well-rested caregiver positively impacts the health and wellbeing of the

4 Improving Ergonomics

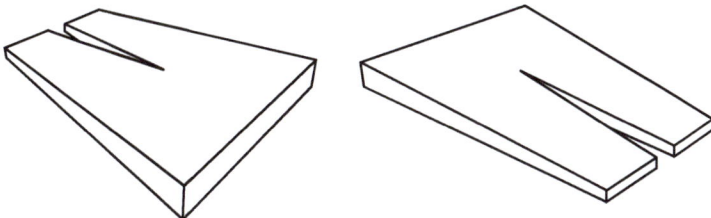

Fig. 4.2 Illustration of the Patented Probax cushion design as viewed from two different angles

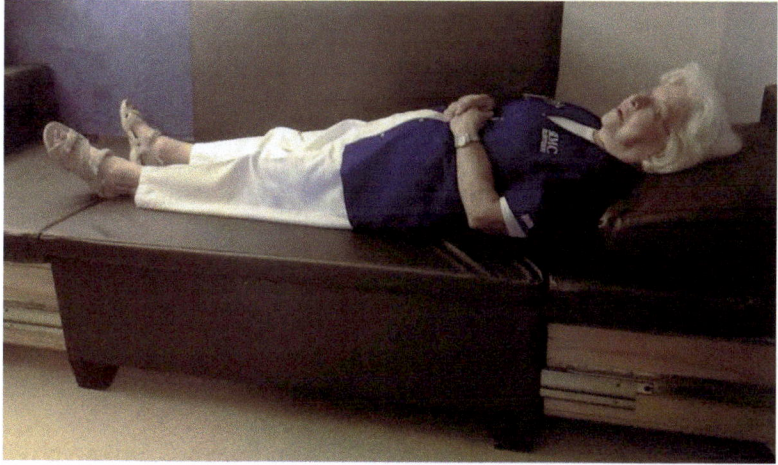

Fig. 4.3 An individual sleeping on the Sit2Sleep furniture

patient for whom they are caring. It is anticipated that the novel Sit2Sleep design (proposed will help caregivers experience better sleep patterns. The Sit2Sleep design is made for comfort, not only during seated activities but more importantly for sleeping. Lastly, the use of a space saving design in the Sit2Sleep will be ideal for smaller hospitals with limited space. The use of the Sit2Sleep furniture by a volunteer at a hospital is shown in Fig. 4.3. The furniture is designed such that it can be easily transformed by moving the arms to the left and right with little effort from a couch meant for sitting to a comfortable bed. The design is wide and long enough (48 in. × 82 in.) to accommodate individuals of varying anthropometric dimensions and aid them in maintaining comfortable sleeping postures.

4.1.3 Goals and Specific Aims

The *long term goal* is to address the issue of health and wellbeing resilience of caregivers. Preliminary data collected from a rural area critical access hospital suggests that the current furniture does not adequately meet the needs of caregivers. The *objective* is to better address the needs of caregivers through furniture design interventions. The *central hypothesis* is that furniture which addresses the needs of caregivers would lead to increased satisfaction and improved health and well-being of caregivers. An intervention through the introduction of a Venous Chair that has shown to improve venous blood flow was examined as part of the solution to better address the needs of caregivers when they perform seated activities. In addition, the novel Sit2Sleep design to better address the needs of caregivers (including family and friends of care recipients) will be examined as part of the solution to address the issue of sleep. The *rationale* for this study is that novel furniture designs which better address the needs of caregivers will result in increased satisfaction, improved health, and, ultimately, resilience in the face of caregiving challenges and risks. The following four specific aims are being proposed:

Specific Aim 1: Determine if the novel Venous Chair designed for caregivers will result in improved caregiver-reported satisfaction. The *working hypothesis* is that the novel Venous Chair will result in higher caregiver-reported satisfaction scores when compared to similar chairs located in the hospital.

Specific Aim 2: Determine if the novel Venous Chair designed for caregivers will result in improved venous blood flow. The *working hypothesis* is that the novel Venous Chair will result in improved venous blood flow in caregivers when compared to a similar chair design currently in use in hospitals.

Specific Aim 3: Determine if the novel Sit2Sleep designed for caregivers will result in improved caregiver-reported satisfaction. The *working hypothesis* is that the novel Sit2Sleep design will result in higher caregiver-reported satisfaction scores.

Specific Aim 4: Determine if the novel Sit2Sleep designed for caregivers will result in improved sleep pattern when compared to current furniture. The *working hypothesis* is that the Sit2Sleep design will result in improved sleep pattern when compared to the current furniture used by caregivers in hospitals.

4.2 Methods

The study was carried out in a rural area hospital in Oklahoma. All the procedures for this study were approved by the Oklahoma State University Institutional Review Board for the protection of human subjects. Twenty individuals were recruited from a rural area hospital.

Specific Aim 1: Determine if the novel Venous Chair designed for caregivers resulted in improved patient-reported satisfaction. The following procedure was followed to address *Specific Aim 1*. The testing procedure involved surveying and interviewing seven individuals in a rural area hospital. Individuals were required to sit on two different chairs: a chair existing in the current hospital and a Venous Chair without ProBax cushion for 30 min each prior to the survey and interview. A survey (see Appendix 1) was conducted with a questionnaire which included general demographic information and 16 Likert-Scale questions (1 = strongly agree, 5 = strongly disagree) to assess the overall satisfaction of the furniture in terms of comfort. Next, an interview was conducted by one of the researchers and included 12 open-ended questions (see Appendix 2) as it relates to the furniture and wellbeing of the individuals in the hospital. Once the data were collected, descriptive and inferential statistics were employed to analyze the data. Key findings (along with quotes) from the interview were documented.

Specific Aim 2: Determine if the novel Venous Chair designed for caregivers resulted in improved venous blood flow. Three caregivers (as part of a pilot study) were asked to sit on two different chairs: a chair existing in current clinic chair and the Venous Chair with ProBax cushion for 30 min each. The caregivers were required to maintain a comfortable, static seated posture. The same posture was maintained while seated on both chairs. At the end of the 30-min period venous blood flow was measured from the popliteal vein using a probe used with an ultrasound machine (Zs3 Zonare ultrasound Doppler equipment). The probe was gently pressed over the skin for 2–3 min to record scans and venous blood flow velocity of the popliteal vein on both left and right limbs of individuals. Once the velocities were recorded the difference in velocities in the two chairs were documented.

Specific Aim 3: Determine if the novel Sit2Sleep designed for caregivers resulted in improved caregiver-reported satisfaction. Surveying and interviewing of seven individuals representative of caregivers in rural area hospitals was conducted while they used the Sit2Sleep furniture. Prior to the survey and interview, researchers explained the different applications of the Sit2Sleep to the caregivers and then they were required to use the Sit2sleep furniture for all the different applications for 45 min. The applications include: sitting, sleeping, and using the side table and the storage. A survey (see Appendix 3) was conducted with a questionnaire which included general demographic information and 18 Likert-Scale questions (1 = strongly agree, 5 = strongly disagree) to assess comfort and ease of use of the furniture. Next, an interview (see Appendix 4) was conducted and included 12 open-ended questions for caregivers as related specifically to caregiver well-being in hospitals. Once the data had been collected, descriptive and inferential statistics were employed to analyze the data collected from the survey.

Specific Aim 4: Determine if the novel Sit2Sleep designed for caregivers resulted in improved sleep pattern. Lastly, three caregivers were recruited for the sleep study using the modified Sit2Sleep prototype. Caregivers were required to wear an actigraphy watch for 7 days. Baseline data was collected for three nights when they slept on beds in the comfort of their own homes. Next, one night of sleep data was collected when they slept on a regular chair that is currently in place in patients' rooms and one night when caregivers slept on the Sit2Sleep furniture. Sleep efficiency while sleeping on the three different pieces of furniture was recorded from the actigraphy watch data.

4.3 Results

In terms of the Venous Chair usability test results in seven individuals ($n = 7$, age: 70.57 years ± 15.13), 100% of the individuals felt comfortable, 85.71% felt (a) relaxed, (b) rested, and (c) that the furniture was spacious, while 71.43% felt that

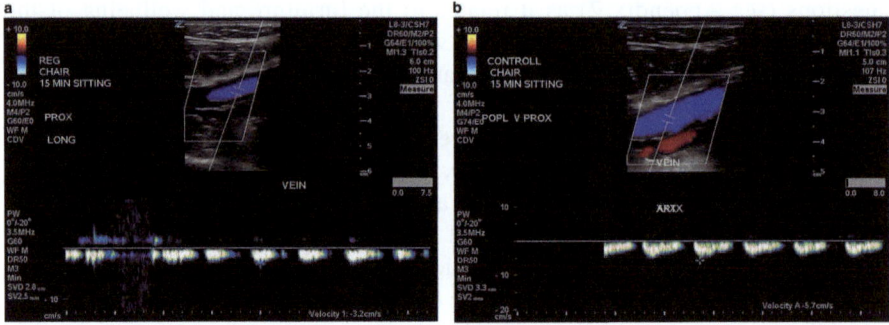

Fig. 4.4. Venous Blood flow scan for (**a**) Clinic Chair and (**b**) Patient Chair

the Venous Chair had even pressure distribution while they sat on it. Venous blood flow data (from the popliteal vein) collected for the left and right limbs (averaged across two trials) for three individuals (age: 67 ± 26.15 years, height = 1.68 ± 6.39 m, weight = 76.06 ± 9.97 kg) showed an average improvement of 10.82% for the left limb and 8.64% for the right limb when individuals sat on the Venous Chair when compared to a regular chair that exists currently in the clinic. Sample venous blood flow data for the clinic chair (with a resulting velocity of 3.2 cm/s) and the Venous Chair (with a resulting velocity of 5.7 cm/s) are shown in Fig. 4.4.

Next, the usability of the Sit2Sleep design based on data from seven (7) individuals (age: 58.00 years ± 17.01) showed that 100% of the individuals found that the Sit2Sleep design was (a) easy to transform, (b) spacious and (c) served multiple purposes. Seventy-one percent (71%) of the caregivers found the Sit2Sleep to be (a) comfortable and (b) visually appealing. However, 42.86% of the individuals reported feeling uneven pressure. In addition to the qualitative data, sleep data collected from three individuals (age: 67 ± 26.15 years, height = 1.68 ± 6.39 m, weight = 76.06 ± 9.97 kg) showed that sleep efficiency was 92.73% when sleeping on their own bed, 57.22% when sleeping on the Sit2Sleep furniture and 34.53% when sleeping on the regular chair currently in the patient rooms. It must be pointed out that this data was not collected from family caregivers of patients but volunteers who are representative of caregivers. Though the Sit2Sleep design appears to help caregivers rest better, there is clearly a need to collect additional data using actual caregivers.

4.4 Discussion

4.4.1 Limitations of the Intervention Designs

Data collected in a rural area hospital showed that the comfort level of the Venous chair was significantly higher when compared to the current chair in the clinic. However, not enough width of the chair for sitting was expressed as a concern. In addition, it was observed that region behind the knee of a short stature individual was making contact with the cushion which might have resulted in a lower venous blood flow. This clearly demonstrates that there is a critical need to look at anthropometry of individuals to determine if there is a good fit between the chair and the individual using it. Buttock-to-knee (popliteal region) length, hip breadth and shoulder breadth could be important measures to consider in design. Alternative chair designs which are wider, broad enough at the shoulders and a design with the front end folding down approximately 80% of the current depth will be examined depending on the cost and feasibility of prototyping new designs.

Data collected from preliminary studies suggest that while the Sit2Sleep does save space and can be easily transformed when a caregiver wants to seep, there were concerns for a better locking mechanism. A sound locking mechanism would prevent the side arm from sliding to the side while the caregiver is seated. In addition, thought the depth of the Sit2Sleep furniture is appropriate to serve as a bed, this could negatively affect the sitting posture of caregivers' with shorter stature. Thus an additional cushion and/or foot rest would be needed to ensure that a caregiver can sit on the Sit2Sleep and maintain optimal sitting posture. Additionally, hospital administrators pointed out that a quality coating of lacquer is needed so that the furniture can be easily cleaned to reduce the passing of infection from one individual to another. Lastly, it was found that the durability of the Sit2Sleep design should be tested so that it can withstand a load of up to 500 lb.

Breakout Box 4.1 Focus on Practice
The experience for caregivers in hospitals or facility-based care settings is commonly primitive and stressful. Caregivers feel responsible for their loved ones; all they want is for their person to be cared for. Hospitals often see outside caregivers as liabilities and additional work for their staff. Professional care teams sometimes forget that informal caregivers (family members and friends) provide crucial social support for the patient which improves patient emotional health and potentially physical health as well. It is critical that caregivers be viewed as assets. They help ensure that patients do not "slip through the cracks" and they serve as the primary care team once the patient leaves the hospital. Caregivers are not properly cared for in healthcare facilities as they are not the priority individuals. Caregivers resort to sleeping upright in chairs, where sleep often does not happen, and resting in uncomfortable environments. A loved one in a hospital puts their caregivers in crisis mode. A lack of adequate rest or restorative sleep will only compound the negative consequences of this situation. How is a caregiver supposed to remember all of the instructions from the healthcare team, instructions which are often laden with medical jargon and complicated routines, when they are not properly rested or thinking clearly? Caregivers need more resources in the hospitals, resources such as improved quality of the accessories in hospital rooms and training for patient care after discharge. More technologically advanced resources for caregivers often translate into more expenses for hospitals, which do not interest them. Improvements need to be cost effective to be considered, but the payout from these improvements can be dramatic. A caregiver who is comfortable and well rested will be paramount to recovery of their loved one.
—Jessica Allen and Mickey Hinds, LIFE Senior Services

4.4.2 Implications

There is a critical need and a clear rationale for addressing the needs of caregivers as those needs related to sitting and sleeping. There is a dearth of literature regarding this topic. Addressing the challenges that caregivers face through design and training interventions is essential for promoting their health and wellbeing. If caregivers are sitting while maintaining a good posture and also getting adequate sleep, they are more likely equipped to better care for a patient. What needs to be considered is how this might be implemented in practice, and, more importantly, how these design interventions play a role in the context of family resilience.

4.4.2.1 Implications for Practice

As pointed out earlier in the chapter, it is estimated that 43.5 million Americans provide care for an individual over the age of 50, and this number will continue to grow with our population ages (Giovannctti & Wolff, 2010). There are individuals of all ages who need care when they are not in good health. Often, the focus is on the needs of the patient, while neglecting the needs of the caregiver. This holds true for hospital administration and practitioners, but more importantly for the family caregivers themselves. There is the assumption that family caregivers will step up and step in as primary service providers, taking on roles that a hospital administrator or practitioner would play (Bailey & Gordon, 2016). As a result, family caregivers take on the responsibility of caring for their loved ones without caring for themselves.

How can design interventions be introduced while educating the different practitioners and administrative personnel in hospital settings as it relates to sitting and sleeping? One of the approaches is to use empathic design (Niinimaki & Koskinen, 2011). If the different practitioners and administrative personnel in hospitals step into the lives of caregivers they would better understand the challenges that caregivers face. If these individuals learn how to care for patients while trying to maintain a good posture and also practice good sleep habits then there is a possibility that they may place a bigger emphasis on the health of caregivers too. In addition, when these individuals experience the comfort resulting from ergonomic design interventions such as the Venous Chair and Sit2Sleep furniture, when compared to existing furniture in their hospitals, they will likely adopt this new technology to help improve the health and wellbeing of caregivers.

In terms of the caregivers, emphasizing the importance of maintaining their health in order to be able to better care for their patients is crucial. In terms of seated activities, along with the design intervention such as the Venous Chair that helps venous blood flow, education on proper sitting and posture is essential. A simple checklist to follow periodically during the day, perhaps in 15-min intervals, is to ensure that the hips, knees and ankles are all in neutral posture. Neutral posture is when the hips, knees and ankles are all at 90°. Excessive deviation from the 90° rule is also not recommended for the elbows. The wrist should be maintained in a neutral posture (equivalent to laying your hand flat on a table) without too much flexion/extension and/or radial/ulnar deviations. Some general guidelines on sitting (Kroemer, 1989) are presented below:

1. **Seat Height**: The seat should be adjustable in height. The minimum range should accommodate the 5th percentile female (30.5 in.) to the 95th percentile male (38.1 in.) as presented in the anthropometric data reported by Kroemer (1989). A good seat height is when the thighs of a caregiver are horizontal, lower legs are vertical, and feet are flat on the floor.
2. **Seat Width**: The seat width should be set to be suitable for larger individuals. A smaller individual can always be accommodated in a larger chair. A width of at least 20 in. is recommended given that the 95th percentile female has a hip breath of 17.2 in. (Kroemer, 1989).
3. **Seat Depth:** The depth should be set to be suitable for shorter individuals. Seat depth should be approximately 20 in. (5th percentile female buttock to knee distance is 20.4 in. while seated; Kroemer, 1989). The importance of an appropriate seat depth is to ensure that all potential caregivers find support in the lumbar area from the backrest. If the seat is any deeper than the thigh length of the shortest person, the front edge of the seat will restrain caregivers from causing their lumbar area to curve to reach the backrest. In addition, the pressure sensitive area at the back of the knee will be pressed against the seat. Accommodating the shortest person is essential in this case because taller caregivers will only suffer from a protruding knee.
4. **Seat Angle**: To provide good seating posture, the seat pan should tilt back approximately 5° to shift the upper torso weight to cause the torso to rest fully against the seat back. This would also prevent caregivers from sliding off the chair. The angle between the seat pan and the seat backrest must be about 105° to keep the torso against the backrest, yet not force the caregivers to lean their head forward in order to balance it properly.
5. **Cushioning**: Cushioning helps distribute the pressures on the ischial tuberosities and on the buttocks caused by the caregiver's weight. This is important because if the pressure is not relieved, discomfort and fatigue will result in the caregivers. Cushioning also allows the body to adopt a stable posture. The cushion thickness should be in the range of 1.5–2 in. The cushion should also not be too soft because after a while this type of seat will become uncomfortable and it will not provide adequate support. It must be pointed out that the cushion used in the Venous Chair has a unique wedge shape design that allows for individuals to maintain a more upright posture, and thereby improve their venous blood flow.

While sitting in a good posture and understanding seating mechanics is essential, it could result in static loading of the back muscles. Thus, it is very important for caregivers to get up and walk every 30 min if they have to sit for long periods of time.

Sitting and sleeping are thus essential to caregiver health and wellbeing. With ergonomic interventions such as the Venous Chair and the Sit2Sleep furniture, and training on good sitting posture and sleep hygiene, caregivers can take care of their health simultaneously while caring for the patients/care recipient.

4.4.2.2 Implications for Family Resilience

For families to be resilient, the health and wellbeing of each individual in the family needs to be considered. A family systems perspective suggests that risk impacting one member of the system impacts all other members and subsystems (see Henry, Hubbard, Struckmeyer, & Spencer, this volume). As caregivers take care of their patients to help them "bounce back", it is vital that they do so without compromising their own health. Patients are often taught to overcome adversity. Caregivers need to do the same. While mental health challenges should be addressed through counseling, this should be combined with simple design interventions and training on physical wellbeing too. Family resilience involves reciprocal dynamics. If a care recipient cannot cope with adversity, the caregiver's health could also be negatively affected. Similarly, when a caregiver cannot cope with adversity, the care recipient's health could be compromised. Thus, if the goal of a caregiver is to help a patient bounce back and have better physical and mental health, the caregiver should keep in mind that the health of the caregiver has a defining role in this process. While there are several dimensions to health and wellbeing of caregivers, simple approaches such as sitting right and sleeping well along with ergonomics design interventions can play a large role in the health and wellbeing of caregivers.

4.4.3 Conclusion

Preliminary results from the study indicate that the Venous chair and the Sit2Sleep furniture designs have positive impacts on seated and sleep related activities. In terms of future directions, an extensive evaluation of the Venous Chair and Sit2Sleep designs should be carried out in different hospital and clinic settings to test for intended use of the furniture by caregivers. The studies would be designed to assess comfort and improvements in blood flow and sleep patterns among caregivers. Successful completion of the project at these different locations could lead to eventual use of the Venous Chair and Sit2Sleep by different hospitals and clinics in the United States to better address the needs of and promote resilience for caregivers.

Questions for Thought and Discussion

1. Is it essential to have ergonomic interventions to better address the needs of caregivers? Will novel design interventions alone result in caregivers sitting and sleeping better? Discuss the importance of educating caregivers to sit and sleep better in combination with ergonomic interventions to help improve their health and wellbeing.
2. What are some of the limitations with the ideas presented in this chapter? What other factors of caregiving are important in your opinion? Briefly discuss.
3. *For health practitioners, health science and human science students*: Develop a sleep guide to help caregivers sleep better so that their health is not compromised while they take care of patients.

4. *For ergonomists and designers*: Develop alternative designs to the Venous Chair and Sit2Sleep furniture to better address the needs of caregivers
5. Create and write a 1–2 page story that is fun and easy to read for a caregiver using a fictional character who has developed low back pain over time as a result of not sitting properly while taking care of a loved one. The story should also be educative so that caregivers who read this story alter their sitting pattern if they are not sitting correctly.
6. Create another story (just like in *Question 5*) but this time with the emphasis on sleeping better.

Appendix 1: Survey for Use with the Venous Chair

Please complete this questionnaire. Your name will not be included with this questionnaire, so your responses are completely <u>confidential</u>. Please circle the number and/or write your responses.

1. Age
2. Gender:
3. Ethnicity:
4. How long does it take for you to come to the hospital?
5. How long are you expected to stay in the hospital during this visit?
6. What is the reason for your hospital visit?

Based on your experience after using the Venous Chair, please answer the following questions:

(1) Strongly agree, (2) Agree, (3) Neutral, (4) Disagree, (5) Strongly disagree

Description	1	2	3	4	5
1. I have sore muscles					
2. My back hurts					
3. I feel stiff					
4. I feel tired					
5. I feel pain					
6. I feel numb					
7. I feel uneven pressure					
8. I feel cramped					
9. I feel relaxed					
10. I feel refreshed					
11. I feel restful					
12. I feel pleased					
13. I feel comfortable					
14. I feel the furniture is spacious					
15. I feel the furniture is visually appealing					
16. I like the furniture					

Appendix 2: Interview Questions After Using the Venous Chair

1. What are your overall impressions of the furniture?
2. What was your impression of the material of the furniture?
3. If you had to give the furniture a grade, from A to F, where A was outstanding and F was very poor, what grade would you give the furniture?

    (a) Why would you give the furniture this grade?

4. What did you like best about the furniture?
5. Was there anything you found less appealing about the furniture?
6. Raise any critical incidents observed when the individual was seated on the furniture —explore as much as possible one incident at a time: What were the actions that you think led up to the incident? What was the problem? How did you try to resolve it? What were you thinking at that time? etc.
7. Did you find similarities or differences between this piece of furniture and others you have used in the past?
8. Are there features you would like to see added to the furniture? If so, what?
9. If you could suggest one change to this furniture, what change would you suggest?
10. Would you consider using this furniture in the future? _____ Why/why not?
11. Would you recommend this furniture to a friend or relative? _____ Why/why not?
12. Do you have any other questions or comments based on your experience with the furniture?

Appendix 3: Survey for Use After Using the Sit2Sleep Furniture

Please complete this questionnaire. Your name will not be included with this questionnaire, so your responses are completely <u>confidential</u>. Please circle the number and/or write your responses.

1. Age:
2. Gender:
3. Ethnicity:
4. How long does it take for you to come to the hospital?
5. How long are you expected to stay in the hospital during this visit?
6. What is the reason for your hospital visit?

    Based on your experience after using the Sit2Sleep, please answer the following questions:

(1) Strongly agree, (2) Agree, (3) Neutral, (4) Disagree, (5) Strongly disagree

Description	1	2	3	4	5
1. I have sore muscles					
2. My back hurts					
3. I feel stiff					
4. I feel tired					
5. I feel pain					
6. I feel numb					
7. I feel uneven pressure					
8. I feel cramped					
9. I feel relaxed					
10. I feel refreshed					
11. I feel restful					
12. I feel pleased					
13. I feel comfortable					
14. I feel the furniture is spacious					
15. I feel the furniture is visually appealing					
16. I like the furniture					
17. I feel the furniture is easy to transform					
18. I feel the furniture serves multiple purposes					

Appendix 4: Interview Questions After Using the Sit2Sleep Furniture

1. What are your overall impressions of the furniture?
2. What was your impression of the material of the furniture?
3. If you had to give the furniture a grade, from A to F, where A was outstanding and F was very poor, what grade would you give the furniture?

    (a) Why would you give the furniture this grade?

4. What did you like best about the furniture?
5. Was there anything you found less appealing about the furniture?
6. Raise any critical incidents observed when the individual was seated on the furniture —explore as much as possible one incident at a time: What were the actions that you think led up to the incident? What was the problem? How did you try to resolve it? What were you thinking at that time? etc.
7. Did you find similarities or differences between this piece of furniture and others you have used in the past?
8. Are there features you would like to see added to the furniture? If so, what?

9. If you could suggest one change to this furniture, what change would you suggest?
10. Would you consider using this furniture in the future? _____ Why/why not?
11. Would you recommend this furniture to a friend or relative? _____ Why/why not?
12. Do you have any other questions or comments based on your experience with the furniture?

References

Bailey, W. A. & Gordon, S. R. (2016). Family caregiving amidst age-associated cognitive changes: Implications for practice and future generations. *Family Relations*, (65). doi:10.1111/fare.12176.

Castellucci, H. I., Arezes, P. M., & Viviani, A. A. (2010). Mismatch between classroom furniture and anthropometric measures in Chilean schools. *Applied Ergonomics*, *41*, 563–568.

CDC Fact Sheet on the State of Aging and Health in America. (2013). Retrieved January 16, 2015, from http://www.cdc.gov/features/agingandhealth/state_of_aging_and_health_in_america_2013.pdf

Charles Alan. (2015). *ProBax technology in Charles Alan seating*. Retrieved January 9, 2017, from http://www.charlesalaninc.com/probax/

Dahl, R. E., & Lewin, D. S. (2002). Pathways to adolescent health: Sleep regulation and behavior. *Journal of Adolescent Health*, *47*, 479–497.

Dianat, I., Karimi, M. A., Hashemi, A. A., & Bahrampour, S. (2013). Classroom furniture and anthropometric characteristics of Iranian high school students: Proposed dimensions based on anthropometric data. *Applied Ergonomics*, *44*, 101–108.

Ding, J. (2011). Sleep deficit, fatigue, and health in family caregivers of persons with dementia awaiting placement. *Master of Nursing Thesis in Aging*. Edmonton: University of Alberta.

Giovannetti, E. R., & Wolff, J. L. (2010). Cross-survey differences in national estimates of numbers of caregivers of disabled older adults. *The Milbank Quarterly*, *88*, 310–349.

Gouvali, M. K., & Boudolos, K. (2006). Match between school furniture dimensions and children's anthropometry. *Applied Ergonomics*, *37*, 765–773.

Helander, M. G., & Zhang, L. (1997). Filed studies of comfort and discomfort in sitting. *Ergonomics*, *40*, 895–915.

Henry, C. S., Hubbard, R. L., Struckmeyer, K. M., & Spencer, T. A. (this volume). Family resilience and caregiving.

Kroemer, K. H. E. (1989). Engineering anthropometry. *Ergonomics*, *32*, 767–784.

Lee, B., Jung, K., Jeong, J., Kim, J., Hong, W., Park, S., & You, H. (2015). Ergonomic evaluation of console chairs for a weapon locating radar. In *Proceedings of the Human Factors and Ergonomics Society 59th Annual Meeting* (pp. 1409–1413).

Maolne, E. B., & Dellinger, B. A. (2011). *Furniture design features and healthcare outcomes*. Retrieved February 11, 2015, from https://www.healthdesign.org/sites/default/files/FurnitureOutcomes_2011.pdf

Mittermayr, M., Fries, D., Gruber, H., Peer, S., Klingler, A., Fischbach, U., … Schobersberger, W.(2007). Leg edema formation and venous blood flow velocity during a simulated long-haul flight. *Thrombosis Research*, *120*, 497–504.

Molenbroek, J. F. M., Kroon-Ramaekers, Y. M. T., & Snijders, C. J. (2003). Revision of the design of a standard for the dimensions of school furniture. *Ergonomics*, *46*, 681–694.

Niinimaki, K., & Koskinen, I. (2011). I love this dress, it makes me feel beautiful! Empathic knowledge in sustainable design. *The Design Journal: An International Journal of all Aspects of Design*, *14*, 165–186.

O'Keeffe, M., Dankaerts, W., O'Sullivan, P., O'Sullivan, L., & O'Sullivan, K. (2013). Specific flexion-related low back pain and sitting: Comparison of seated discomfort on two different chairs. *Ergonomics, 56*, 650–658.

Oyama, H., Ebine, Y., Ando, T., & Noro K. (2004). Measurement of venous blood flow in the lower limbs: Prevention of deep vein thrombosis during prolonged sitting. In *Proceedings of the International Conference WWCS, Kuala Lumpur* (Vol. 7, pp. 302–305).

Rashid, M., & Zimring, C. (2008). A review of the empirical literature on the relationship between indoor environments and stress in healthcare and office settings: Problems and prospects of sharing evidence. *Environment and Behavior, 40*(2), 151–190.

Trochelman, K., Albert, N., Spence, J., Murray, T., & Slifcak, E. (2012). Patients and their families weigh in on evidence based hospital design. *Critical Care Nurse, 32*, e1–e11.

Chapter 5
Hope as a Coping Resource for Caregiver Resilience and Well-Being

Chan M. Hellman, Jody A. Worley, and Ricky T. Munoz

In 2015, there was an estimated 43.5 million unpaid adult caregivers in the U.S. representing 18.2% of the total population. Indeed, 3.7 million of these adults provide care for children with 33.3 million providing care for another adult. A majority (85%) of care recipients are family members with approximately one-half reporting they had no choice in their role as caregiver (National Alliance for Caregiving & AARP, 2015). To be certain, caregiving can result in a rewarding experience for both the caregiver and recipient. Nevertheless, the existing research on caregivers has focused on the negative outcomes often manifesting from a sense of burden and psychological stress (Schulz, Visintainer, & Williamson, 1990). Indeed, the NAC/AARP (2015) report shows that 40% of the informal caregivers are in high burden situations with another 25% reporting moderate burden. Because of the potential burden and strain associated with caregiving, these unpaid adult providers are at a higher risk for emotional, social, and health related difficulties (Vitaliano, Zhang, & Scanlan, 2003).

Caregiving burden and stress has been shown to have negative health consequences with higher rates of illness, disease, and use of prescription medication (Haley et al., 1995; Kiecolt-Glaser, Dura, Speicher, Trask, & Glaser, 1991; Kipp, Nkosi, Laing, & Jhangri, 2006; Soskolne, Halevy-Levin, & Ben-Yehuda, 2007;

C.M. Hellman, Ph.D. (✉)
College of Arts and Sciences, University of Oklahoma, Tulsa and OU Center of Applied Research for Nonprofit Organizations, 4502 East 41st Street, Tulsa, OK 74135, USA
e-mail: chellman@ou.edu

J.A. Worley, Ph.D.
OU Department of Human Relations and Center of Applied Research for Nonprofit Organizations, 4502 East 41st Street, Tulsa, OK 74135, USA
e-mail: jworley@ou.edu

R.T. Munoz, J.D.
Anne and Henry Zarrow School of Social Work and OU Center of Applied Research for Nonprofit Organizations, 4502 East 41st Street, Tulsa, OK 74135, USA
e-mail: munoz@ou.edu

Vitaliano et al., 2003). Caregivers report higher levels of anxiety, depression, anger, and dysfunctional coping (Del-Pino-Casado, Perez-Cruz, & Frias-Osuna, 2014; Leggett, Zarit, Kim, Almeida, & Klein, 2015; Schulz, O'Brien, Bookwala, & Fleissner, 1995; Zarit, Orr, & Zarit, 1985). Caregivers are also more likely to report isolation from social support networks (George & Gwyther, 1986; Hoppes, Bryce, Hellman, & Finlay, 2012) and an increase in family-work conflict (McDaniel & Allen, 2012). Evidence suggests that care recipients are at an increased risk for lower levels of care, abuse, and hospitalization when the caregiver is suffering from the negative effects of burden and stress (Beach et al., 2005).

Given the prevalence of unpaid caregiving in the U.S. and the potential negative consequences associated with burden and stress for both the caregiver and recipient, efforts are needed to facilitate resilience among caregivers by enhancing their capacity to positively cope with adversity and contribute to their potential to flourish. A growing body of research associated with the positive psychology movement points to the psychological strength of hope as an important coping resource that has particular relevance to caregiver resilience. This chapter introduces the positive psychology construct of hope within the context of Snyder's (2002) theoretical model and the empirical literature supporting its importance as a coping resource. Finally, we present an integration of hope as a resilience process within the context of caregiving.

5.1 Positive Psychology

For much of the twentieth century, identifying, preventing, and treating dysphoria, a state of unease or dissatisfaction with life, dominated the field of psychology. However, the introduction of positive psychology in the last 15 years has unified scholars toward the scientific study of strengths that enable individuals, groups, and institutions to thrive (Seligman & Csikszentmihalyi, 2000). One major premise of the positive psychology philosophy is that these measurable strengths can serve as buffers (i.e., protective processes) protecting individuals from adversity and stress. Seligman's (2011) recent conceptualization of well-being theory argues that 24 character strengths are paramount in the ability to flourish. He argues that when we are in situations that allow us to fully utilize our strengths, we are more likely to be engaged, experience positive emotions and find meaning in the pursuit of goals, and have more positive relationships. These 24 character strengths are clustered within six virtues (Wisdom and Knowledge, Courage, Humanity, Justice, Temperance, and Transcendence) that are universally understood and valued, as well as measurable. It is beyond the scope of this chapter to review these character strengths in detail. However, the interested reader should consider the works of Christopher Peterson (cf. Peterson & Seligman, 2004).

Hope is a character strength within the virtue of Transcendence and is empirically connected to this evolving perspective of positive psychology. For instance, Feldman and Snyder (2005) argued that hope is an important component to

5 Hope as a Coping Resource

understanding the meaning we attribute to our experience as we pursue our desired goals. Henry, Morris, and Harrist (2015) highlight meaning-making as one of the significant family adaptive systems that facilitate resilience. Feldman and George & Gwyther, 1986 Snyder's study found that when controlling for hope, the relationships between meaning and well-being are diminished. Hope also contributes positively to an individual's familial and personal relationships. The establishment of positive relationships at an early age tends to relate to higher hope and more meaningful relationships later in life (Westburg, 2001). Empirical studies of the 24 character strengths have found that hope is among the top predictors of well-being across the life span (cf. Park, Peterson, & Seligman, 2004a, 2004b; Peterson, Ruch, Beermann, Park, & Seligman, 2007).

5.2 Hope Theory

Hope is a motivational process that assumes all human behavior is grounded in the expected attainment of a desirable goal. Hope theory advances a long tradition of other psychological expectancy value theories (cf. Bandura, 1977; Lewin, 1951) by articulating the strategies component of goal attainment (Lee, Locke, & Latham, 1989). Lewin articulated the cognitive nature of goal setting from the expectancy of achieving the goal along with the value placed upon the goal. Bandura extended this line of reasoning by introducing the self-efficacy the individual holds toward attaining the specific goal, utilizing available skills and control over the environment. Nevertheless, it is Snyder's (2002) hope theory that articulates and emphasizes the pathways and agency thinking that individuals utilize toward goal attainment (Fig. 5.1).

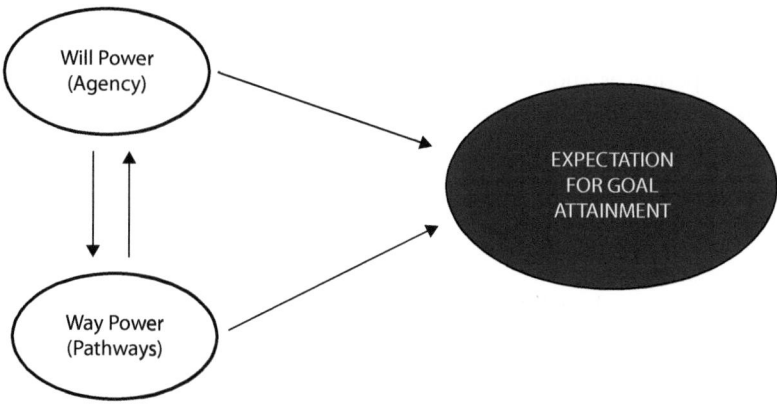

Both pathways and agency are required for hope...agency without pathways is more likely a wish!

Fig. 5.1 Hope theory

Snyder's (2002, 2004) hope model is a cognitive based motivational model of goal attainment. In particular, this model specifies an additive and reciprocal relationship between agency and pathway thinking toward attainment of any desired goal. *Agency thinking* reflects the motivational aspect of hope theory. To the extent that a caregiver can devote mental energy to begin and continue a strategy toward attaining the goal they would be considered agentic. Agentic thinking would require that the caregiver desires the goal as well as believing they had the capacity to pursue, sustain, and achieve the goal (Arnau, Rosen, Finch, Rhudy, & Fortunato, 2007). *Pathway thinking* reflects the ability of the caregiver, a parent for example, to conceive one or more cognitive strategies to goal attainment. High hope caregivers are able to articulate multiple viable pathways toward their goals. Moreover, they are able to develop alternative strategies toward a desired goal when faced with a barrier. Snyder (2002) articulates that individuals with high hope will be confident in their ability to purse their chosen pathway. Hope theory further prescribes that both agency and pathways are necessary components of hope. Any deficit in this cognitive theory (goals, agency, pathways) reflects low hope. Indeed, neither agency nor pathway thinking alone is sufficient to sustain hope. Caregivers must be able to cognitively articulate a goal, consider specific strategies with measurable benchmarks to attainment, and have the mental energy to pursue and maintain the pathway toward the goal. Snyder (1995, 1996) theorized this cognitive process as one that builds upon itself. Achieved success in the creation of plans towards a goal in turn fuels motivation and desire to begin and sustain these plans. Likewise, energized and excited thoughts about a goal in turn encourage thoughts related to planning and strategizing how to achieve the goal. As an example, a caregiver experiencing burden and stress could decide to learn mindfulness as a self-care strategy. Identifying self-care as a desirable goal, will increase the mental energy (agency thinking) needed to consider and pursue the goal. With agency thinking enhanced, the caregiver is primed to search for strategies of self-care (pathways thinking). While there may be multiple potential strategies, the caregiver determines that mindfulness is a viable pathway relative to their likely time constraints. As the caregiver experiences short-term success in in their well-being, mental energy is fueled to continue practicing or perhaps try new mindfulness strategies.

5.3 Significance of Hope

The research is clear: hopeful people are more likely to be resilient and flourish than low hope people. Hopeful individuals are able to identify productive paths towards reaching their identified goals, manage and overcome stress, and report lower levels of daily stress (Chang, 1998; Irving, Snyder, & Crowson, 1998; Ong, Edwards, & Bergeman, 2006; Snyder, 2002). Overall, the experience of hope has a positive influence on individual health and well-being (Gallagher & Lopez, 2009; Shorey, Little, Snyder, Kluck, & Robitschek, 2007; Snyder et al., 1996). Magaletta and Oliver (1999) reported that individuals with high hope experience better overall physical, psychological, and social well-being. Hope is linked to more positive and less negative affect (Snyder et al., 1991; Steffen & Smith, 2013); overall life satisfaction (Bailey, Eng, Frisch, & Snyder, 2007; Valle, Huebner, & Suldo, 2004); perceived physical health (Wrobleski & Snyder, 2005); and overall life meaning and sense of purpose (Feldman & Snyder, 2005; Mascaro & Rosen, 2005; Michael & Snyder, 2005). Hopeful people have also been found to be less reactive to stressful situations (Chang & DeSimone, 2001; Snyder, 2002). Indeed, the development of agency and pathway thinking serve as a cognitive skill set that could potentially bolster a caregiver's ability to move towards the utilization of resources that enable resiliency (Snyder, Feldman, Taylor, Schroeder, & Adams, 2000). In terms of coping strategies, hope is positively associated with engaged coping and negatively associated with avoidant coping (Chang & DeSimone, 2001; Roesch, Duangado, Vaughn, Aldridge, & Villodas, 2010). Hope interventions also reduce depression, hopelessness, and anxiety in psychiatric populations (Cheavens et al., 2005; Klausner et al., 1998). In sum, the evidence suggests that the tenets of hopeful thinking can be leveraged to improve emotion regulation, well-being, meaning making, relationship building, and achievement. To be sure, hope is a fundamental component of our capacity to thrive and a critical resource to caregivers in potential high burden and stress environments.

5.4 Hope Is Not Self-Efficacy or Optimism

To further understand the meaning of hope, it is helpful to consider hope in relation to selected other constructs that bear resemblance. Both self-efficacy and optimism are similar to hope and deserve attention to distinguish their meanings.

5.4.1 Self-Efficacy

Bandura (1986) defines self-efficacy as the perceived confidence individuals have about their capacity to pursue and attain a specific goal. Snyder (2000) acknowledges similarities between the states of hope and self-efficacy. However, Snyder notes important differences. First, hope contains an agency dimension that parallels self-efficacy (i.e., "I can do this"), but also contains the willingness to *initiate* and *sustain* movement toward goals "I will do this" and "I am doing this". As such, hope involves cognitive elements that extend beyond appraisals of self-efficacy. While Bandura also advances a hope pathways-like construct, known as outcome expectancies, Bandura consistently deemphasizes outcome expectancies' value to other outcome variables of well-being (Bandura, 1986). In contrast, while Bandura holds self-efficacy as the driver of goal pursuit, hope theory places equal emphasis on both hope agency and hope pathways cognitions (Snyder, 2000). Research supports empirical distinctiveness between traditional measures of self-efficacy and hope in contributing to wellbeing outcomes (Magaletta & Oliver, 1999; O'Sullivan, 2011).

5.4.2 Optimism

Much as hope shares similarities with self-efficacy, hope also has commonalities with optimism. Optimism theory has two main variants, one that involves an optimistic attribution style (Seligman, 1991) and the other viewing optimism as a generalized expectancy for success (Scheier & Carver, 1985). While hope shares similarities with both formulations of optimism, hope remains distinct. Seligman's optimism theory (1991) makes the attribution process central to optimism, meaning that when an individual experiences negative life events, such as failure to achieve goals, the optimistic person attributes the failure to external forces that are variable and specific instead of to internal, stable, and global causes. The importance of achieving goals to well-being is implicit in the optimistic attribution style, as the optimistic person is effective at distancing himself/herself from failure. Despite the similarities between this view of optimism and hope in that both hold the value of goal attainment as central to wellbeing, Snyder's view of hope is distinct, for when a person has higher levels of hope, that individual takes the "next step" by moving beyond the initial act of distancing oneself from past failures toward actively approaching desired goals (Snyder, 1994). Hope is also distinct from Schieer and Carver's view (1985) that optimism is a general expectancy that goals will be achieved. In this understanding of optimism, the expectancy of a positive outcome is seen as the primary driver of goal (engaging/disengaging) pursuit behavior. Hope, while sharing similarities to this formulation of optimism in that both involve expectancies of future goal attainment, hopeful thinking involves cognitive appraisals including both the desire for a positive outcome (agency) and the appraisal of the pathways one has to reach those goals. Thus, when both agency and pathways are present, the two domains iteratively generate greater overall hope (Snyder, 1994).

5.5 The Loss of Hope

Those who have experienced repeated failure when attempting to achieve their goals are likely to be aware of their deficits in pathways and agency capacity. Those low hope individuals will face goals with a focus on failure and experience negative emotional responses (e.g., anger, sadness, despair). Repeated failed attempts to achieve desirable goals can result in the loss of hope (Fig. 5.2). Indeed, the loss of hope is a process that deserves attention. When we recognize that we do not know how to achieve our desired goals, and when faced with significant barriers with no perceived viable alternative paths, the first phase in the loss of hope is *rage*. While high hope individuals can often identify alternative pathways as a coping response,

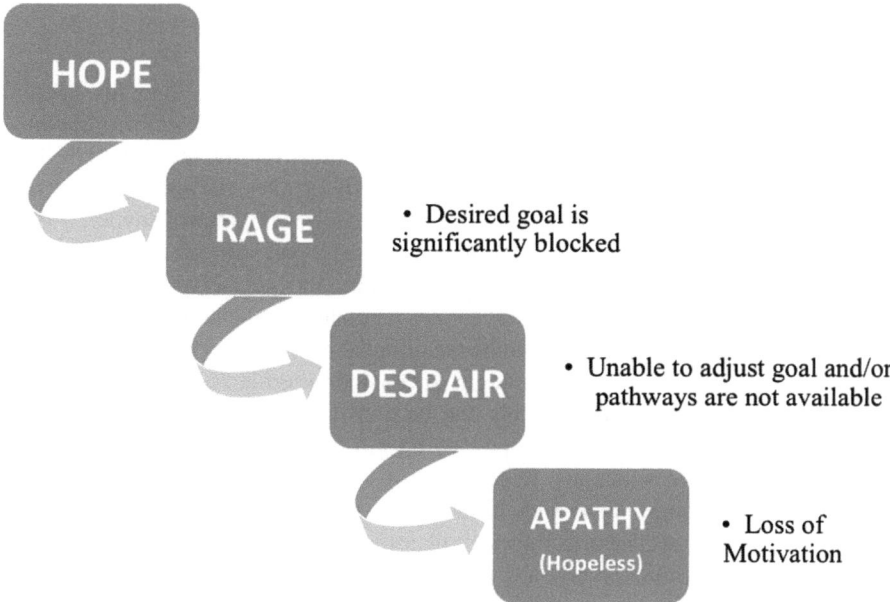

Fig. 5.2 The loss of hope

the demise of hope is based upon the loss of viable pathways toward a highly desirable goal resulting in the immediate experience of rage (an intensely focused negative cognition/emotion). The second phase of hopelessness is *despair*. This occurs when viable alternatives are no longer available or the individual is unable to adjust their goal. In this condition, the barriers to goal attainment are recognized as insurmountable and the individual questions the meaning and value of their efforts. Because the goal remains desirable, requiring mental energy, the individual is experiencing the loss of hope due to the lack of viable pathways but is not yet hopeless as they continue to direct mental energy (agency) toward their object of desire. The final phase in the loss of hope is *apathy*. The goal is seen as unobtainable thus no mental energy is expended in considering the desirability of the goal let alone the potential pathways that must be considered. Indeed, apathy is often characterized as a lack motivation and goal-directed thoughts and behavior (Marin, 1990; Reekum, Stuss, & Ostrander, 2005) and therefore clearly the opposite of hope. Interestingly enough, some caregiver research exists to suggest that apathy is associated with distress and depression resulting from the loss of functioning required for caregiving (cf. Reekum et al., 2005).

5.6 Nurturing Hope

While the previous section described the process of diminishing hope, this section will focus on how hope can be nurtured (Fig. 5.3). To start, the desirable goal must be described in specific detail and exist within the realm of possible attainment. This initial stage of *goal clarification* tends to temporarily increase the agency dimension of hope allowing for a parallel focus on pathways development (Snyder, 1995). Next, *viable pathways* to goal attainment can be developed with enough attention to detail to allow for measurable benchmarks. Benchmarks can serve as an important feedback system allowing individuals to self-regulate their behavior and emotions. Within this stage, individuals should be encouraged to consider potential barriers to their chosen pathways so they can begin to consider alternative pathways or detail strategies to overcome barriers. This can be a critical time in nurturing hope, as those who have experienced low hope may be still focused on the potential for failure and demonstrate reluctance to continue on the pathway to hope. Next, is the phase of *creating future memories*. In this stage, the individual will reflect on how success will feel, consider how they will be impacted and how they will behave. In this stage, the individual creates a realistic image of success. This process of creating future memories serves to reinforce mental energy (i.e., agency). As the individual approximates the desirable goal, their agency and pathways thinking should be elevated reflecting higher hope. Furthermore, successful goal attainment allows the now hopeful individual to pursue related goals and further develop a trail style of hope.

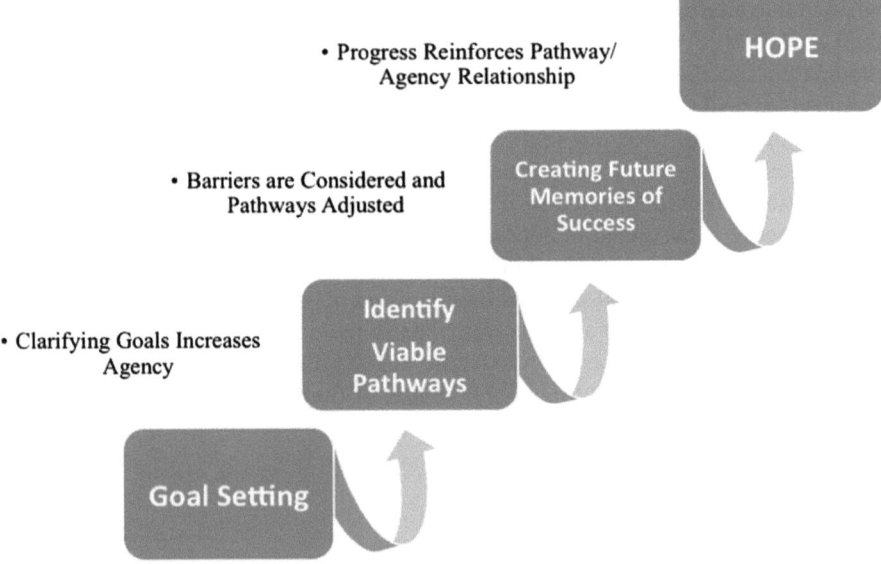

Fig. 5.3 Nurturing hope

5.7 Hope and Caregiving

Protective factors that promote resilience and hope are likely to create opportunities for family caregivers to maintain a positive outlook and find meaning and purpose in their role. Following a review of research about families and cancer, Jones (2012) concluded that most parents do seem to adjust and cope with the circumstances around having a child with cancer, but that a significant majority of parents experience symptoms characteristic of post-traumatic stress. Jones also noted the disruption to identity and structure among families where there is a shift to parenting a child with cancer. These disruptions were found to contribute to negative outcomes for the caregivers. Strategies (pathways) that might reduce long-term distress include individuals sharing hope by maintaining a positive demeanor (Hinds et al., 2009) or by providing direct and forthcoming information for caregivers (Maurer et al., 2010).

Parental caregiving takes on additional dimensions when a child is facing the end of life. Caregiving in that context might involve balancing the hope for a cure with the devastating reality that the child is likely to die (Jones, 2012). This reference to "hope for cure" in the context of caring for a sick child is not the cognitive process that Snyder conceptualized as dispositional hope, with desirable goals, viable pathways, and individual agency. In fact, high mental energy (e.g., arousal, focus, motivation) toward a desirable outcome with no viable pathway is more likely a wish rather than hope. When faced with insurmountable barriers to the goal (e.g., terminal illness), hopeful caregivers are likely to engage in re-goaling (Snyder, 2002). For instance, recent studies have shown that parents want to be seen as a "good parent" to their critically ill or dying child (Hinds et al., 2009; Maurer et al., 2010). In the language of hope, this is evidence of a desirable goal adjusted from a previously blocked goal. This goal or desire to be seen as a "good parent" is a powerful internal motivator of decision-making and actions (Hinds et al., 2009). This internal motivation is an aspect of what hope theory recognizes as agency.

Experiencing a hopeful perspective in general might be a way that families involved in the care of a member with a chronic illness stay psychologically healthy (Robinson, 2001). In fact, Venning, Eliot, Whitford, and Honnor (2007) demonstrated that self-efficacy and depression scores predicted the hope levels among caregivers of children with chronic illness. Because the relationship between a caregiver and child with a chronic illness is reciprocal, a caregiver's level of hope is important to the child (Seren Cohen, 1999). Low hope among parents of a child with chronic illness might hinder their ability to provide a sense of safety for the child (Venning et al., 2007).

5.8 Hope and Resilience Among Caregivers

Darlington and Bland (2002) stressed the importance of the family and health workers as "hope carriers" (i.e., pathways) when the patient has experienced repeated unsuccessful goal pursuits. This assertion can be extended to the hopefulness among family caregivers of those patients. It is reasonable to expect that sources of hope can function to increase the resilience among family caregivers in coping with the stress associated with providing care for a physically or mentally ill family member. Bland and Darlington (2002) found that hope was an integral part of a family's ability cope, and that hope contributes to a more positive future orientation and positive expectations.

Not only is it important that the family members experience hope, but the mode of projecting hope towards the ill family member may be even more important. This projection of hope is particularly challenging in the context of perceived caregiver burden. Hernandez, Barrio, and Yamada (2013) observed that an increase in hope was associated with decreased caregiver burden. Moreover, the observed contribution of hope to decreased caregiver burden exceeded the effects explained by the diagnosed family member's length of illness and severity of symptoms. Hope was also found to be a stronger predictor of adaptation than perceived uncertainty among family caregivers (Truitt, Biesecker, Capone, Bailey, & Erby, 2012).

Hope enables a caregiver to maintain involvement with a family member, and continue seeking adequate caregiving opportunities (Bernheim, Lewine, & Beale, 1982) even when others might not be optimistic. Similarly, Flaskas (2007) describes how families affected by stress or trauma might balance feelings of hope and hopelessness by shifting from one to the other in relation to the level of hope among other family members. For example, a primary caregiver within a family may fall into feelings of hopelessness while other caregivers within the same family may rally a sense of hope, with feelings of hope and hopelessness changing as events unfold. This type of dynamic illustrates how a systemic view of the family may be more helpful in understanding resilience processes (Henry et al., 2015). Clearly, a better understanding of the interplay between hope and resilience has important implications for caregiver well-being.

5.9 Implications: Evidence-Informed Strategies for Fostering Hope and Resilience Among Family Caregivers

There is no universal list of effective strategies for recovery or protective factors for family caregivers. However, a review of recent research and literature recognizes common salient attributes among resilient, healthy families. These factors include: a positive outlook, spirituality, family member accord, flexibility, communication, time together, routines and rituals, and social support (Black & Lobo, 2008; Harrist, Henry, Liu, & Morris, in press; Olson, 2000; White, Richter, Koeckeritz, Munch, & Walter, 2004). When taking on the role of caregiver, the experience of burden and strain may challenge these important protective factors leaving the caregiver vulnerable for psychological, physical, and social difficulties.

Breakout Box 5.1 Implications for Practice
We'd only been married for about a year when my wife shared with me the good news that she was pregnant with our first child. About that same time, I received a once-in-a-lifetime offer to work part time for a church in Louisiana, and study at a local university. So we packed everything we owned into a couple of suitcases and moved from Venezuela to the US with just enough savings to buy an old car and our first bed. The pregnancy wasn't easy. My wife had never been to the US and all the new smells and flavors made her nauseous all the time. In fact, nothing was easy: we couldn't get insurance because the pregnancy was a pre-existing condition; the little house we could afford to rent only had one small window unit in the bedroom for AC; I started classes and work, and my wife, who spoke no English, was home alone with not so much as a TV to keep her company. Still, we had our hopes and dreams, which turned the challenges into an opportunity to deepen our bond as a couple as we prepared for the arrival of our baby.

Finally, the day arrived. After 17 long, hard hours of labor and the help of the dreaded "Pitocin Drip" our son made his grand entry into the world. Unfortunately, what should have been a moment of joy-filled relief, was only the beginning of raging storm. Nurses quickly whisked our baby away as my wife, literally delirious from the ordeal of giving birth, was given a sedative and put under. Sometime later, I was quickly informed that our son was born hypoglycemic, had some cardiac issues, and most likely had a syndrome of some kind based on several patterned anomalies. How bad? We would know more after the specialists examined him. I was stunned and understood little of what was said. At that point a terrifying thought rushed into my brain: How would I tell my wife that she cannot hold her baby?!

The NICU was a learning experience on steroids. We sat by my son's incubator as specialists of every brand marched in with their distinct train of students talking, pointing, and concurring. My son began to look like a pin cushion as the nurses struggled to find another place to draw blood for yet another round of testing. After 11 days, the pediatric cardiologist said my son had a small heart murmur that was nothing to worry about, and the geneticist couldn't find a diagnosis that fit. So, my son, now able to eat on his own was—or so we thought—deemed stable enough for us to take home.

Being home didn't last long. My son wasn't eating, couldn't eat. After another 6 weeks in a hospital, my son was diagnosed with a severe heart condition that was inoperable due to him being too weak to survive surgery (the syndrome growing ever more apparent remained elusive and undiagnosed). Once again we were sent home, but this time it was different. We were placed into hospice care. The doctors gave him about 2 weeks to live. The most likely

(continued)

Box 5.1 (continued)

scenario was that he would catch any little bug, which would lead to pneumonia, which then would cause him to drown in his own fluids. They were partially correct. Over the next 4 years he developed pneumonia five times plus a couple of other illnesses along the way. Each time he was not expected to live, but he did! Finally, we found a surgeon who would operate and attempt to fix his heart. That was 26 years ago.

Now, when I look back, I wonder how my wife and I made it? How did our marriage not only stay together, but get stronger? How did I finish a Master's degree in the midst of everything else that was going on? How were we able to be in and out of hospitals, caring for a dying child during four long years, and still maintain our sanity? I think the answer is found in the hope that comes from a strong faith and in being part of a community of folks that shares and nurtures that hope. Regardless of what happened to our son, my wife and I always knew, ultimately, where we were going, and the path that was going to get us there. We were convinced that even during the darkest hours of making funeral preparations, when death seemed eminent, there was purpose and meaning in everything that happened. We didn't understand and we didn't like our situation, but we decided to trust and believe. When we were emotionally overwhelmed and unable to fight any longer, we were surrounded by others who supported us and kept us standing by the power of their faith. Having this hope allowed us to maintain a semblance of normality in our life. At about the 2-year mark of my son's odyssey, God blessed us with another child—a beautiful healthy little girl. She, too, gave us strength as we determined to make life as normal as possible for her.

Life has not always been easy. Even after the surgery that gave my son a new opportunity on life, he is still severely multiply impaired, and still without a diagnosis. As a result of complications associated with his condition, he has been in and out of hospitals his entire life, each time staring death in the face. Now, however, we consider him to be our family's biggest blessing. He has taught us so much and enriched our lives in ways unimaginable. The research literature seems to always focus on the stress and burdens that accompany caring for a special needs child. People often seem to look at us with either sympathy or compassion, grateful that they have healthy children. And although I wouldn't wish the pain we have experienced on anyone, I would like to, 1 day, write a book detailing all the wonders entailed in being a caretaker; even when the one for whom we care is teetering on death.

All of us eventually go through difficult times. To be able to withstand life's toughest storms, it is paramount to find your unmovable rock, that fortress of beliefs and convictions that map out the path you are to take even in the darkest of times; to hold to them with an unwavering and tenacious hope; and to become part of a community that nurtures and sustains your hope when you are too weak to make it on your own. If you are a caregiver, it is my prayer that you, too, will find your rock and that your hope will sustain you when the night falls.

—Caleb's dad.

5.9.1 Implications for Practice and Policy

Although the role of caregiver for a family member presents a unique context for uncertainty and strain, there is evidence to suggest that these circumstances do not necessarily result in a life that feels overwhelming and burdensome (Lefley, 1997). Caregiving can sometimes have all the features of a chronic stress experience when accompanied by high levels of uncertainty and unpredictability (Schulz & Sherwood, 2008). Ambiguity and uncertainty can have a significant effect on stress and anxiety. However, the cognitive-based motivational process of identifying desirable goals and selecting among alternative pathways (i.e., hope) can help regulate what the caregiver feels and does, and therefore alleviate a sense of uncertainty or feeling a loss of control. Less ambiguity exists when self-regulation is employed as a means of control because it provides cognitive structuring. Individual caregivers can have hope and feel capable of expanding their personal abilities and making their own choices despite uncertainty and ambiguity. This process of fostering hope in the face of adversity may be mediated by cognitive and communication processes (Redlich, Hadas-Lidor, Weiss, & Amirav, 2010).

For example, proposed areas of intervention with patients and caregivers in the context of clinical nursing include encouraging teamwork and mutual support to increase family bonds and decrease stress; fostering open communication to increase understanding and feelings of connectedness; and encouraging self-care to maintain physical and emotional resources of the caregivers (Northouse, Katapodi, Schafenacker, & Weiss, 2012). Family members who have a relative with serious mental illness experienced significant increases in hope after they received an intervention designed to positively alter cognitions in family members (Redlich et al., 2010). The mediated learning approach in that intervention focused on teaching family members about cognition and how it relates to everyday functioning combined with training of communication skills from a meditative perspective (e.g., intentional sharing and access to knowledge generally held by professionals; Redlich et al., 2010).

5.9.2 Implications for Understanding Family Resilience

Froma Walsh (2003, 2006) suggests several ways that resilient families handle adversity. She agrees that linking with resources and empowering beliefs enable families to better cope with stress (Walsh, 2012) and her work highlights the importance of clear and consistent communication within families (Walsh, 2003, 2012). This is particularly important for caregiving families who face multiple challenges. Based on her extensive research and clinical work with families, Walsh identifies nine family processes that support resilient families (Rolland & Walsh, 2006; Walsh, 2003, 2006) consistent with previous research, which has generally defined family resilience in terms of individual, family, and community factors (Coyle et al., 2009; Greeff, Vansteenwegen, & Ide, 2006).

5.10 Conclusion

Taking on the role of caregiver, while potentially rewarding and meaningful, is likely to be associated with burden and strain that can impact one's goals and desires. Hope represents an emerging conceptual framework that can have significant benefit to the study of caregiver well-being and resilience. Caregivers who have the opportunity to consider one or more pathways toward their goals will have a higher likelihood of thriving in their role. Additionally, the ability to direct and maintain mental energy (agency) toward goal pursuits will help reduce the burden and strain typically associated with caregiving. Strategies that enhance both pathways and agency among caregivers will advance coping resources especially important during difficult and stressful experiences (Cicchetti, 2013; Meaney, 2010; Rolland & Walsh, 2006).

Questions for Thought and Discussion

1. Discuss the three dimensions of hope theory (goals, pathways, agency) to ensure the language of hope is clearly understood. Ask each group member to describe caregiving examples where hope is present highlighting goals, pathways, and agency.
2. Discuss how a caregiver might loose hope using the stages of hopelessness. How might this theory explain caregiver maltreatment behaviors?
3. Using a hypothetical caregiving scenario, differentiate hope from optimism and self-efficacy.
4. Compare caregiver hope as it relates to acute and long-term care.
5. Describe hope, self-efficacy and optimism as it relates to caregiver well-being. In this discussion, compare how these psychological strengths are both similar and different.
6. Consider a hypothetical situation in which a new caregiver believes their desired goals are no longer viable since they imagine themselves constrained by their new role. Discuss strategies using pathways and agency in which hope can be nurtured for this caregiver.
7. Research suggests that willpower (agency) is a finite resources associated with glucose levels in the blood. What are the implications to caregiving in terms of self-care?
8. Given the definition of hope used in this chapter, how might a caregiving parent who "hopes for a cure" in a terminally ill child be considered false hope? Is this illusionary process bad?

References

Arnau, R. C., Rosen, D. H., Finch, J. F., Rhudy, J. L., & Fortunato, V. J. (2007). Longitudinal effects of hope on depression and anxiety: A latent variable analysis. *Journal of Personality, 75*, 43–64.

Bailey, T. C., Eng, W., Frisch, M. B., & Snyder, C. R. (2007). Hope and optimism as related to life satisfaction. *Journal of Positive Psychology, 2,* 168–175.

Bandura, A. (1977). *Social learning theory.* Englewood Cliffs, NJ: Prentice Hall.

Bandura, A. (1986). *Social foundations of thought and action: A social cognitive theory.* Englewood Cliffs, NJ: Prentice-Hall.

Beach, S. R., Schulz, R., Williamson, G. M., Miller, L. S., Weiner, M. F., & Lance, C. E. (2005). Risk factors for potentially harmful informal caregiver behavior. *Journal of the American Geriatrics Society, 53,* 255–261.

Bernheim, K. F., Lewine, R. R., & Beale, C. T. (1982). *The caring family: Living with chronic mental illness.* New York, NY: Random House.

Black, K., & Lobo, M. (2008). A conceptual review of family resilience factors. *Journal of Family Nursing, 14,* 33–55.

Bland, R., & Darlington, Y. (2002). The nature and source of hope: Perspectives of family caregivers of people with serious mental illness. *Perspectives in Psychiatric Care, 38,* 61–68.

Chang, E. C. (1998). Hope, problem-solving ability, and coping in a college student population: Some implications for theory and practice. *Journal of Clinical Psychology, 54,* 953–962.

Chang, E. C., & DeSimone, S. L. (2001). The influence of hope on appraisals, coping, and dysphoria: A test of hope theory. *Journal of Social and Clinical Psychology, 20,* 117–129.

Cheavens, J. S., Rosenthal, M. Z., Daughters, S. B., Nowak, J., Kosson, D., Lynch, T. R., & Lejuez, C. W. (2005). An analogue investigation of the relationships among perceived parental criticism, negative affect, and borderline personality disorder features: The role of thought suppression. *Behaviour Research and Therapy, 43,* 257–268.

Cicchetti, D. (2013). Annual research review: Resilient functioning in maltreated children—Past, present, and future perspectives. *Journal of Child Psychology and Psychiatry, 54,* 402–422.

Coyle, J. P., Nochajski, T., Maguin, E., Safyer, A., DeWit, D., & Macdonald, S. (2009). An exploratory study of the nature of family resilience in families affected by parental alcohol abuse. *Journal of Family Issues, 30,* 1606–1623.

Darlington, Y., & Bland, R. (2002). The nature and sources of hope: Perspectives of family caregivers of people with serious mental illness. *Perspectives in Psychiatric Care, 38,* 61–68.

Del-Pino-Casado, R., Perez-Cruz, M., & Frias-Osuna, A. (2014). Coping, subjective burden and anxiety among family caregivers of older dependents. *Journal of clinical Nursing, 23,* 3335–3344.

Feldman, D. B., & Snyder, C. R. (2005). Hope and the meaningful life: Theoretical and empirical associations between goal-directed thinking and life meaning. *Journal of Social and clinical Psychology, 24,* 401–421.

Flaskas, C. (2007). Holding hope and hopelessness: Therapeutic engagements with the balance of hope. *Journal of Family Therapy, 29,* 186–202.

Gallagher, M. W., & Lopez, S. J. (2009). Positive expectancies and mental health: Identifying the unique contributions of hope and optimism. *Journal of Positive Psychology, 4,* 548–556.

George, L. K., & Gwyther, L. P. (1986). Caregiver well-being: A multidimensional examination of family caregivers of demented adults. *The Gerontologist, 26,* 253–259.

Greeff, A. P., Vansteenwegen, A., & Ide, M. (2006). Resiliency in families with a member with a psychological disorder. *The American Journal of Family Therapy, 34,* 285–300.

Haley, W. E., West, C. A. C., Wadley, V. G., Ford, G. R., White, F. A., Barrett, J. J., … Roth, D. L. (1995). Psychological, social, and health impact of caregiving: A comparison of Black and White dementia family caregivers and noncaregivers. *Psychology and Aging, 10,* 540–552.

Harrist, A. W., Henry, C. S., Liu, C., & Morris, A. S. (in press). The third wave of family resilience research. In B. H. Fiese (Ed.), *APA handbook of contemporary family psychology.*

Henry, C. S., Morris, A. S., & Harrist, A. W. (2015). Family resilience: Moving into the third wave. *Family Relations, 64,* 22–43. doi:10.1111/fare.12106

Hernandez, M., Barrio, C., & Yamada, A. (2013). Hope and burden among Latino families of adults with schizophrenia. *Family Process, 52,* 697–708.

Hinds, P. S., Oakes, L. L., Hicks, J., Powell, B., Srivastava, D. K., Spunt, S. L., ... Furman, W. L. (2009). 'Trying to be a good parent' as defined by interviews with parents who made phase I, terminal care, and resuscitation decisions for their children. *Journal of Clinical Oncology, 27,* 5979–5985.

Hoppes, S., Bryce, H., Hellman, C. M., & Finlay, E. (2012). The effects of brief mindfulness training on caregivers' well-being. *Activities, Adaptation & Aging, 36,* 147–166.

Irving, L. M., Snyder, C. R., & Crowson, J. J. J. (1998). Hope and coping with cancer by college women. *Journal of Personality, 66,* 195–214.

Jones, B. L. (2012). The challenge of quality care for family caregivers in pediatric cancer care. *Seminars in Oncology Nursing, 28,* 213–220.

Kiecolt-Glaser, J. K., Dura, J. R., Speicher, C. E., Trask, O. J., & Glaser, R. (1991). Spousal caregivers of dementia victims: Longitudinal changes in immunity and health. *Psychosomatic Medicine, 53,* 345–362.

Kipp, W., Nkosi, T. M., Laing, L., & Jhangri, G. S. (2006). Care burden and self-reported health status of informal women caregivers of HIV/AIDS patients in Kinshasa, Democratic Republic of Congo. *Aids Care, 18,* 694–697.

Klausner, E. J., Clarkin, J. F., Spielman, L., Pupo, C., Abrams, R., & Alexopoulas, G. S. (1998). Late-life depression and functional disability: The role of goal-focused group phsychotherapy. *International Journal of Geriatric Psychiatry, 13,* 707–716.

Lee, T. W., Locke, E. A., & Latham, G. P. (1989). Goal setting theory and job performance. In L. A. Pervin (Ed.), *Goal concepts in personality and social psychology.* Hillsdale, NJ: Erlbaum.

Lefley, H. P. (1997). Synthesizing the family caregiving studies: Implications for service planning, social policy, and further research. *Family Relations, 46,* 443–450.

Leggett, A. N., Zarit, S. H., Kim, K., Almeida, D. M., & Klein, L. C. (2015). Depressive mood, anger, and daily cortisol of caregivers on high- and low-stress days. *Journals of Gerontology: Psychological Sciences, 70,* 820–829.

Lewin, K. (1951). *Field theory in social science.* New York, NY: Harper & Row.

Magaletta, P. R., & Oliver, J. M. (1999). The hope construct, will, and ways: Their relations with self-efficacy, optimism, and general well-being. *Journal of Clinical Psychology, 55,* 539–551.

Marin, R. S. (1990). Differential diagnosis and classification of apathy. *The American Journal of Psychiatry, 147,* 22–30.

Mascaro, N., & Rosen, D. H. (2005). Existential meaning's role in the enhancement of hope and prevention of depressive symptoms. *Journal of Personality, 73,* 985–1013.

Maurer, S. H., Hinds, P. S., Spunt, S. L., Furman, W. L., Kane, J. R., & Baker, J. N. (2010). Decision making by parents of children with incurable cancer who opt for enrollment ofn a phase I trial compared with choosing a do not resuscitate/terminal option. *Journal of Clinical Oncology, 28,* 3292–3298.

McDaniel, K. R., & Allen, D. G. (2012). Working and care-giving: The impact on caregiver stress, family-work conflict, and burnout. *Journal of Life Care Planning, 10,* 21–32.

Meaney, M. J. (2010). Epigenetics and the biological definition of gene x envioronment interactions. *Child Development, 81,* 41–79.

Michael, S. T., & Snyder, C. R. (2005). Getting unstuck: The roles of hope, finding meaning, and rumination in the adjustment to bereavement among college students. *Death Studies, 29,* 435–458.

National Alliance for Caregiving and AARP. (2015). *Caregiving in the US.* Retrieved from http://www.aarp.org/content/dam/aarp/ppi/2015/caregiving-in-the-united-states-2015-report-revised.pdf

Northouse, L. L., Katapodi, M. C., Schafenacker, A. M., & Weiss, D. (2012). The impact of caregiving on the psychological well-being of family caregivers and cancer patients. *Seminars in Oncology Nursing, 28,* 236–2245.

O'Sullivan, G. (2011). The relationship between hope, stress, self-efficacy, and life satisfaction among undergraduates. *Social Indicators Research, 101,* 155–172.

Olson, D. H. (2000). Circumplex model of marital and family systems. *Journal of Family Therapy*, 22, 144–167.
Ong, A. D., Edwards, L. M., & Bergeman, C. S. (2006). Hope as a source of resilience in later adulthood. *Personality and Individual Differences*, 41, 1263–1273.
Park, N., Peterson, C., & Seligman, M. E. P. (2004a). Strengths of character and well-being. *Journal of Social and Clinical Psychology*, 23, 603–619.
Park, N., Peterson, C., & Seligman, M. E. P. (2004b). Reply: Strengths of character and well-being: A closer look at hope and modesty. *Journal of Social and Clinical Psychology*, 23, 628–634.
Peterson, C., Ruch, W., Beermann, U., Park, N., & Seligman, M. E. P. (2007). Strengths of character, orientations to happiness, and life satisfaction. *The Journal of Positive Psychology*, 2, 149–156.
Peterson, C., & Seligman, M. E. P. (2004). *Character strengths and virtues: A handbook and classification*. New York, NY: Oxford University Press.
Redlich, D., Hadas-Lidor, N., Weiss, P., & Amirav, I. (2010). Mediated learning experience intervention increases hope of family members coping with a relative with severe mental illness. *Community Mental Health Journal*, 46, 409–415.
Reekum, R. V., Stuss, D. T., & Ostrander, L. (2005). Apathy: Why care? *Journal of Neuropsychiatry and Clinical Neuroscience*, 17, 7–19.
Robinson, J. (2001). Editorial. *Journal of Advanced Nursing*, 34, 567–568.
Roesch, S. C., Duangado, K. M., Vaughn, A. A., Aldridge, A. A., & Villodas, F. (2010). Dispositional hope and the propensity to cope: A daily diary assessment of minority adolescents. *Cultural Diversity and Ethnic Minority Psychology*, 16, 191–198.
Rolland, J. S., & Walsh, F. (2006). Facilitating family resilience with childhood illness and disability. *Current Opinion in Pediatrics*, 18, 527–538.
Scheier, M. F., & Carver, C. S. (1985). Optimism, coping, and health: Assessment and implications of generalized outcome expectancies on health. *Journal of Personality*, 55, 169–210.
Schulz, R., O'Brien, A. T., Bookwala, J., & Fleissner, K. (1995). Psychiatric and physical morbidity effects of dementia caregiving: Prevalence, correlates, and causes. *The Gerontologist*, 35, 771–791.
Schulz, R., & Sherwood, P. R. (2008). Physical and mental health effects of family caregiving. *American Journal of Nursing*, 108, 23–27.
Schulz, R., Visintainer, P., & Williamson, G. M. (1990). Psychiatric and physical morbidity effects of caregiving. *Journal of Gerontology: Psychological Sciences*, 45, 181–191.
Seligman, M. E. P. (1991). *Learned optimism*. New York, NY: Knopf.
Seligman, M. E. P. (2011). *Flourish: A visionary new understanding of happiness and well-being*. New York, NY: Free Press.
Seligman, M. E. P., & Csikszentmihalyi, M. (2000). Positive psychology: An introduction. *American Psychologist*, 55, 5–14.
Seren Cohen, M. (1999). Families coping with childhood chronic illness: A research review. *Families, Systems & Health*, 17, 149–166.
Shorey, H. S., Little, T. D., Snyder, C. R., Kluck, B., & Robitschek, C. (2007). Hope and personal growth initiative: A comparison of positive, future-oriented constructs. *Personality and Individual Differences*, 43, 1917–1926.
Snyder, C. R. (1994). *The psychology of hope: You can get there from here*. New York, NY: Free Press.
Snyder, C. R. (1995). Conceptualizing, measuring, and nurturing hope. *Journal of Counseling and Development*, 73, 355–360.
Snyder, C. R. (1996). To hope, to lose, and hope again. *Journal of Personal and Interpersonal Loss*, 1, 3–16.
Snyder, C. R. (2000). *Handbook of hope: Theory, measures, and applications*. San Diego, CA: Academic Press.
Snyder, C. R. (2002). Hope theory: Rainbows in the mind. *Psychological Inquiry*, 13, 249–275.

Snyder, C. R. (2004). Hope and other strengths: Lessons from animal farm. *Journal of Social and Clinical Psychology, 23*, 624–627.

Snyder, C. R., Feldman, D. B., Taylor, J. D., Schroeder, L. L., & Adams, V. H. (2000). The roles of hopeful thinking in preventing problems and enhancing strengths. *Applied & Preventive Psychology, 9*, 249–270.

Snyder, C. R., Harris, D., Anderson, J. R., Holleran, S. A., Irving, L. M., Sigmon, S. T., ... Harney, P.(1991). The will and the ways: Development and validation of an individual-differences measure of hope. *Journal of Personality and Social Psychology, 60*, 570–585.

Snyder, C. R., Sympson, S. C., Ybasco, F. C., Borders, T. F., Babyak, M. A., & Higgins, R. L. (1996). Development and validation of the State Hope Scale. *Journal of Personality and Social Psychology, 70*, 321–335.

Soskolne, V., Halevy-Levin, S., & Ben-Yehuda, A. (2007). The context of caregiving, kinship tie and health: A comparative study of caregivers and non-caregivers. *Women & Health, 45*, 75–94.

Steffen, L. E., & Smith, B. W. (2013). The influence of between and within-person hope among emergency responders on daily affect in a stress and coping model. *Journal of Research in Personality, 47*, 738–747.

Truitt, M., Biesecker, B., Capone, G., Bailey, T., & Erby, L. (2012). The role of hope in adaption to uncertainty: The experience of caregivers of children with Down syndrome. *Patient Education and Counseling, 87*, 233–238.

Valle, M. F., Huebner, E. S., & Suldo, S. M. (2004). Further evaluation of the Children's Hope Scale. *Journal of Psychoeducational Assessment, 22*, 320–337.

Venning, A. J., Eliot, J., Whitford, H., & Honnor, J. (2007). The impact of a child's chronic illness on hopeful thinking in children and parents. *Journal of Social and Clinical Psychology, 26*, 708–727.

Vitaliano, P. P., Zhang, J., & Scanlan, J. M. (2003). Is caregiving hazardous to one's physical health? A meta-analysis. *Psychological Bulletin, 129*, 946–972.

Walsh, F. (2003). Family resilience: A framework for clinical practice. *Family Process, 42*, 1–18. doi:10.1111/j.1545-5300.2003.00001.x

Walsh, F. (2006). *Strengthening family resilience*. New York, NY: Guilford Press.

Walsh, F. (2012). Family resilience: Strengths forged through adversity. In F. Walsh (Ed.), *Normal family processes* (pp. 399–427). New York, NY: Guilford Press.

Westburg, N. G. (2001). Hope in older women: The importance of past and current relationships. *Journal of Social and Clinical Psychology, 20*, 354–365.

White, N., Richter, J., Koeckeritz, J., Munch, K., & Walter, P. (2004). "Going Forward": Family resiliency in patients on hemodialysis. *Journal of Family Nursing, 10*, 357–378. doi:10.1177/1074840704267163

Wrobleski, K. K., & Snyder, C. R. (2005). Hopeful thinking in older adults: Back to the future. *Experimental Aging Research, 31*, 217–233.

Zarit, S. H., Orr, N. K., & Zarit, J. M. (1985). *The hidden victims of Alzheimer's disease*. New York, NY: New York University Press.

Chapter 6
Voices from Down Home: Family Caregiver Perspectives on Navigating Care Transitions with Individuals with Dementia in Nova Scotia, Canada

Emily Roberts

Dementia is a term used to describe a group of diseases which cause a progressive decline in the ability to think, speak, remember, and carry out normal daily activities. As of 2015, 47.5 million people worldwide were living with dementia and that global number is expected to increase to an estimated 75.6 million in 2030 (Alzheimer's Association, 2015).

Past studies have found that family members with a relative with dementia often experience what has been called the 'unexpected career of caregiver' and face multifaceted, complex, and stressful life situations that have important consequences (Raina et al., 2004). While these individuals may be motivated to provide care out of a sense of love or reciprocity, spiritual fulfilment, a sense of duty, guilt, or social pressures (Brodaty & Donkin, 2009), the impact of dementia on the family member in its advanced stages resembles having lost a spouse or parent, as the person with dementia may lose the ability to speak and may no longer recognize family members (Abby, Froggard, Parker, & Abby, 2005). Multiple factors make the adjustment to the caregiving role particularly hard, as the caregiver balances this role with other demands, including child rearing, career, and other relationships (Connidis, 2010).

Increasing dependency on government resources in older populations and the high cost of long term care (LTC) have resulted in families being encouraged to provide home-based care for as long as possible, resulting in an increasing disparity between service requirements, user involvement, and service provision (Bramble, Moyle, & McAllister, 2009). Family caregivers are often referred to as "in-formal" caregivers to distinguish them from paid caregivers like nurses and aides. The term informal suggests casual, unstructured, unofficial care, yet these individuals carry out medical tasks that if performed by a nurse would be considered skilled care. This categorization ignores demanding medical tasks, frequent lack of cooperation

---

E. Roberts, Ph.D. (✉)
Department of Design, Housing, and Merchandising, College of Human Sciences, Oklahoma State University, 437 Human Sciences, Stillwater, OK 74078, USA
e-mail: emily.roberts12@okstate.edu

from care recipients with dementia, constant strain of managing behavioral disturbances, as well as the financial and managerial challenges of caregiving over long periods of time (Levine, Halper, Peist, & Gould, 2010).

Despite these factors, making the decision to relinquish the caregiving to health care providers can be a very difficult and stressful event (Caron & Bowers, 2003). Many family caregivers have made significant personal sacrifices to keep their family members at home (Park, Butcher, & Mass, 2004), and have often developed important patterns of coping, mastery, and hardiness over the course of their family caregiving role (Gaugler, Kane, & Newcomer, 2007).

6.1 Caregiver Resilience

In order to withstand these challenges, the long-term nature of dementia caregiving requires long-term support strategies that are oriented around various transitions that merge in the context of the caregiving career (Gaugler, Pot, & Zarit, 2007). Navigating any health system can be difficult, and a lack of coordination across health systems and settings can create barriers for those trying to access appropriate care and service for their family member across that continuum of care. Therefore, the constructs of self-mastery, self-efficacy, hopefulness, acceptance, and stress resistance become necessary components of a caregiver's coping capabilities and this construct is often referred to as resilience. Caregiver resilience may be termed as the use of successful coping strategies by informal and formal caregiver, shifting from a burden perspective which heavily saturates the literature to a resilience perspective (Ross, Holliman, & Dixon, 2003).

A consistent theme in dementia caregiving research is the diversity of responses to care demands and one potentially predictive factor in caregiver adaptation to that role is resilience (Gaugler, Pot, & Zarit, 2007). Resilience as a psychological conceptualization is the ability to maintain normal or enhanced functioning during times of adversity (Cherry et al., 2013), and consists of two components. The first is thriving and succeeding and the second is exhibiting this competence in difficult situations or a situation where others often do not succeed. Walsh (2003) describes a family resilience model of adaptation which includes making meaning out of adversity, having a positive outlook, spirituality, flexibility, and connectedness with each other and the community.

Resilience in dementia caregiving may account for diversity in outcomes over time, depending on various levels of perceived burden (i.e., high or low burden) in the presence of various levels of care demands (i.e., high or low care demands). Gaugler, Pot, & Zarit, (2007) suggest that resilience in dementia caregiving is part of a dynamic self-regulatory process that is influenced by the occurrence of different environmental stressors and is also composed of a series of intrapsychic dimensions that may or may not respond to changes in care-related stressors over time. They go on to point out that resilience is influenced by three constellations of variables: context of care; the status of the care recipient; and individual, family and community resources.

Resistance to stress from caregiving roles may take the form of coping and resilience, yet over the continuum of care and a sustained depletion of resources, caregivers may be at risk themselves for declines in physical and cognitive health without an adequate support system (Fig. 6.1). Families represent the bridge between the time and place that have been left behind and the present day (Chaudhury, 2002), therefore the deeply rooted, long-term relationship between the caregiver and his or her family member is an important area of study in order to understand the impact of care transitions over time on both caregiver and care recipient well-being (Strang, Koop, Dupuis-Blanchard, Nordstrom, & Thompson, 2006). When studying caregiver responses in care transitions, it is important to look at the impact of societal and cultural expectations on the caregiving experience, values and preferences of the individual caregivers, positive aspects of caregiving, and the history and quality of the care receiver/caregiver relationship (Feinberg, Newman, Gray, & Kolb, 2004; Guberman, 2005). Therefore, the objective of this qualitative study—part of a larger study exploring the provincial continuing care system in Nova Scotia, Canada—was to examine the experiences of family caregivers through the course of the four transition nodes of dementia diagnosis, home care, trauma/event, and a permanent move to LTC.

6.2 The Continuum of Care

The behavioral and psychological symptoms that are core features of Alzheimer's disease and related dementias include a cluster of neuropsychiatric symptoms such as depression, apathy, sleep disorders, agitation, and psychosis. Individuals with dementia may have multiple psychological, biological, and interpersonal unmet needs, as they lose their grasp of understanding of their circumstances and rely heavily on their family member's for all aspects of their physical and emotional support, as well as activities of daily living (Geda et al., 2013). The most common form of dementia is Alzheimer's disease, which makes up more than 64% of all cases. Other types of dementia include vascular dementia, vascular dementia due to stroke, dementia of the Lewy body type, Parkinson's disease, Picks disease, and Huntington's disease (Nova Scotia Department of Health and Wellness, 2015).

The nature of the dementia care challenge is therefore varied and individuated, calling attention to the need to address each circumstance within the broader life context. Because of the long-term trajectory of dementia, the role changes for family caregivers prior to LTC are subtle and at times insidious with varying degrees of detrimental physical and emotional impacts for family members (Bramble et al., 2009) Although resilience appears to be present in dementia caregiving and may account for diversity in outcomes over time, few efforts have attempted to conceptualize resilience directly across the continuum of dementia care (Gaugler, Pot, & Zarit, 2007). Therefore, while there is currently much research related to the predictors of institutionalization, it is also important to gain greater insight into caregiver experiences throughout the continuum of care in order to provide more appropriate and sensitive support through this journey (Gaugler, Leach, Clay, & Newcomer, 2004).

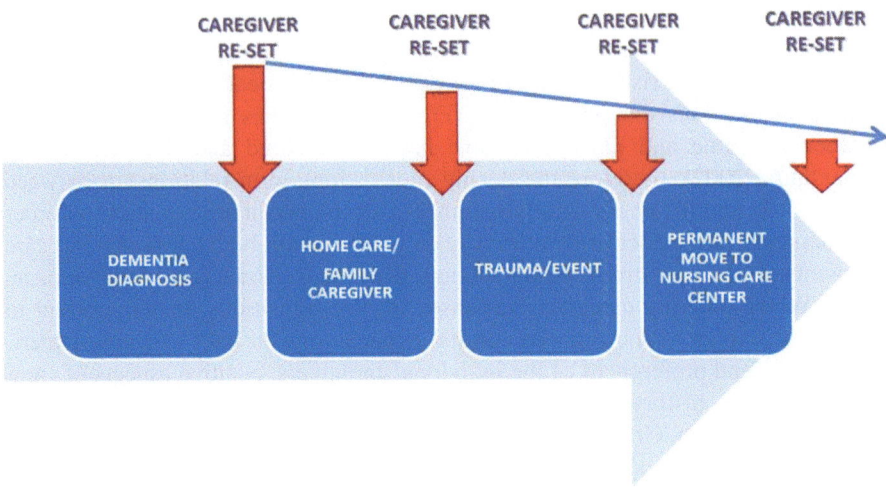

Fig. 6.1 Trajectory of resilience through the continuum of care

6.3 Care Transitions

The deeply rooted, long-term relationship between the caregiver and his or her family member, whether it be positive or negative, is fundamental to understanding the caregiver experience through the continuum of care, starting with home care after an initial dementia diagnosis (Strang et al., 2006). Buhr, Kuchibhatla, and Clipp (2006) identified the relative importance of factors which were evident in the year prior to nursing home placement and which served as reasons for the placement decision. These reasons were examined and correlated with indicators of caregiver and care recipient physical and emotional functioning, with principle predictors being (a) the need for more skilled care, (b) the caregiver's health, (c) the care recipient's dementia-related behaviors, and (d) the need for more assistance.

While still at home, individuals with dementia may be living with serious chronic illnesses which lead them to cycle in and out of emergency departments or hospitals numerous times (Levine et al., 2010). Care planning under these circumstances can be piecemeal, and when care needs change, transitions can be ineffective and stressful for both the caregiver and care recipient. Caregivers may also be unaware of the deterioration of the person with dementia until there is crisis, usually a hospitalization of the person for a medical problem that finally alerts the caregiver to the cognitive decline. Families may experience exhaustion, deep sorrow, or fractured relationships as they make a decision to place a family member into LTC (Strang et al., 2006). In addition, once the decision has been made for a transition to long term care, caregivers may experience a trying time of waiting and transitions.

Gaugler, Pot, et al. (2007) describe two effects that care placement may have on caregivers once their relative is admitted into a care facility. One possibility is that prolonged stress associated with ongoing care and seeing one's relative continue to

> **Breakout Box 6.1 Implications for Practice**
> As a seasoned attorney whose work has focused for 37 years in the area of estate planning and guardianship, I will share what I have witnessed to be the biggest predictors of an individual's ability to successfully cope with the demands of caring for a loved one with dementia. In many ways, this type of caregiver role is like a dance. It is a dance in which you have multiple leading partners and you are trying to shift the style and steps of your dance to your leading man. Education, organization, and support are critical, but the most important thing is to have a sense of humor. When a person has dementia, the possibilities of what may happen are endless. As a result, caregivers must be educated about the aging process and must be willing to learn about the disease itself. The more educated the fewer surprises there will be, and more surprises lead to greater stress levels. If you are educated about the disease you are better equipped to deal with it. Second, there has to be a schedule of who will help and when. You cannot have a situation where one person is a full time caregiver without any sort of relief. Keep in mind that it is easy for family members to lose their compassion and kindness, which is an issue that is rarely discussed. This type of caregiving can be an "icky" job and it is never ending, so there has to be relief – both for the caregiver and the victim of the disease.
> —Ms. Robyn Owens, Managing Partner, The Owens Law Firm, P. S.

decline would result in deterioration in the caregiver's resources and well-being. In contrast to this wear and tear model, it is possible that caregivers will adapt and become more resilient over time, learning new coping strategies or distancing themselves emotionally from their relative.

Research supports the notion that families often continue to hold responsibilities and in many instances provide direct care as they transition from being primary caregiver, with total responsibility for looking after their family member, to now watching care staff in a facility do those same activities (Keefe & Fancey, 2000). Family caregivers may play an important role in encouraging and supporting therapeutic goals, providing comfort and reassurance, and becoming care monitors and advocates (Levine et al., 2010). Caregivers typically want their family members to be treated like they had been at home, therefore retaining some measure of control is linked to a family member's desire for their loved one to be treated with dignity and respect within the institution (Strang et al., 2006). Often, tension between LTC care staff and families is a reflection of the staff not fully recognizing this unchanging nature of the caregiver dyad, therefore care staff may help families through these transitions through open communication, offers of education, and opportunities to involve families in care of their family members (Maas et al., 2004).

6.4 Continuing Care in Nova Scotia

Through each of the discussed care transitions, family caregivers often remain vigilant advocates for the well-being of their family member with dementia, expending emotional and physical resources along the way. The healthcare system in Nova Scotia, Canada, has one of the few legislated policies in place geared specifically to address the needs of family caregivers and care recipients throughout the continuum of care. Referred to by many simply as "down home", Nova Scotia is the one of the poorest of the Canadian provinces and is roughly the geographical size of the state of West Virginia and the population of the state of Delaware. The population of less than a million people often require and depend on government assistance in a number of areas, and one primary area of need is healthcare.

Of the ten Canadian provinces, Nova Scotia has the highest proportion of people aged 65 and over (17.7% in 2013) and one of the fastest aging populations. Today, more than 17,000 Nova Scotians are living with dementia and that number is expected to double by the year 2038 with estimates that a resulting 2.5% of the population will be living with Alzheimer's disease and related dementias. It is projected that from 2008–2038 Nova Scotia will spend over $24.5 billion in direct health costs, unpaid caregiver costs, and indirect costs. This has implications for families, caregivers, and for the health and social system (Nova Scotia Department of Health and Wellness, 2015).

As with the other Canadian provinces, the health care in Nova Scotia is funded by the federal health care system referred to as "national" health insurance. This is a predominantly publicly financed, privately delivered system, based on an interlocking set of provincial and territorial health insurance plans. The system provides access to universal, comprehensive coverage for medically necessary hospital, in-patient, and out-patient physician services. All principal/territorial hospital and medical insurance plans are linked through adherence to national principles set at a federal level, and the management and delivery of health services is the responsibility of each province or territory (Banerjee, 2009).

6.4.1 The Continuing Care Strategy

According to the Canadian Institute for Health Information (CIHI), caregivers of people with dementia provide 75% more care then other caregivers (Nova Scotia Department of Health and Wellness, 2015). The Health Council of Canada notes that in 2012, 2.7 million Canadian family caregivers over the age of 45 were helping seniors with long term health conditions. Three quarters of caregivers were aged 45–64, while one quarter were seniors themselves.

In an attempt to address these statistics, the provincial Department of Health and Wellness (DHW) in Nova Scotia has used funding from the federal health care system to develop a provincial care strategy which includes systems and supports in home health, family caregiving and care transitions across the continuum of care. This Continuing Care Strategy (Nova Scotia Department of Health and Wellness, 2006) is a strategy which addresses care for individuals with physical and cognitive needs and their family members, in order to provide a strong system and network to create smooth transitions for caregiver and care recipients.

Through this system, all forms of home and institutional long term care resources in Nova Scotia are centralized through the Single Entry Access System. This allows individuals or family members to call a central number to request that DHW do a financial and care assessment to determine the level of care necessary and the most appropriate type of care options for an individual with long term care needs, including dementia care. This assessment is required in order to receive any subsidized home aide or nursing home services in the province.

6.4.2 Research Questions

While the aim of the Nova Scotia CCS is to provide support to individuals with dementia and their family caregivers, issues of long wait times, poorly planned transitions, and caregiver concerns for the long term well-being of the family members remain. Participants in the current study described their experiences during their relative's move into LTC, providing insight into an oftentimes confusing and frustrating journey within the provincial continuing care system, while at the same time describing their resilience in the trajectory of their changing roles. Within the context of the provincial CCS designed to provide support for individuals with physical and cognitive needs and their families, the research questions in this study include:

1. What are the relations between burden and resilience for family caregivers living at home with individuals with dementia?
2. Once a determination has been made that a transition to LTC must be made, how do family caregivers experience the wait and transition times within Nova Scotia Continuing Care System?
3. Following a transition of a family member with dementia into LTC, what are the psychological factors involved for family member relinquishing their caregiving roles?

6.5 Methodology

6.5.1 Study Sites

The two study sites for this research were located outside of Halifax, the capitol of Nova Scotia. Ridgemont Continuing Care Center had a resident population of 48 at the time of the study and Stonebridge Continuing Care Center had a resident population of 49. Both sites have a special care unit for individuals with dementia. At Ridgemont, the number of residents with dementia in the locked memory care wing was 12 and at Stonebridge, the number of residents with dementia in the locked household for memory care was ten.

6.5.2 Study Design

In many qualitative studies, inquirers collect multiple forms of data and spend a considerable amount of time in the natural setting (Creswell, 2009). In this study, a total of 8 weeks were spent in the two facilities, and the principle methods of data collection were participant observation and pre-arranged family caregiver interviews. The time in the two communities was equally divided during the two-month period. The majority of weekdays were spent in both communities, as they were about a 20-min drive from one another, although there were some occasions when an entire day was spent at one community. In addition to the interviews and observations, a detailed review of the provincial Continuing Care Strategy and other Canadian Health Care policy documents took place.

6.5.2.1 Interviews

Humans are meaning makers; meaning is identified through experience. Qualitative interviewing is one of the best ways of coming to understand meaning through examining experience (Rubenstein, 2002). In this particular study, face-to-face interviews were conducted with family caregivers of individuals currently living at one of the two study sites. Interviewees were made aware by care staff at the two nursing facilities that the study was taking place though a letter sent out to family members. At Ridgemont, the number of family caregiver interviews conducted was $N = 4$ (female spouse, male spouse, daughter caregiver, son caregiver). At Stonebridge, the number of interviews conducted was $N = 4$ (female spouse caregiver, male spouse caregiver, daughter caregiver, son caregiver) (Table 6.1).

An interview protocol was used for all interviews, which included the following components: a heading defining the date, place, interviewer, and interviewee; the questions beginning with a general questions followed by probing questions that asked individuals to explain their ideas in more detail or elaborate on that they have said. All interviews were pre-arranged with the interviewee and facility administrators and were audio-recorded, and lasted approximately 30–45 min.

Table 6.1 Residents with dementia and their family member

Resident/family member	Resident age	LTC community	Family member theme/resident transition to care
Tom/wife Joan	87	Ridgemont	*He calls me 10–12 times a day* • Moved from hospital after broken hip and pneumonia
Rose/husband Garney	82	Ridgemont	*I'm not moving her again* • Moved from another nursing home due to progressive dementia
George/son John	82	Ridgemont	*He doesn't really know we're here* • Moved from son's home due to progressive dementia
Frank/daughter Tina	82	Ridgemont	*Caring for two parents* • Moved from hospital after pneumonia due to rummaging and danger to himself due to progressive dementia
Richard/daughter Carmen	80	Stonebridge	*They sent him to the wrong nursing home* • Moved from hospital after car accident
Terry/husband Gill	67	Stonebridge	*She's well cared for* • Moved from Ridgemont, need for 24 h physical assistance
Vincent/wife Elizabeth	89	Stonebridge	*There's a limit to what you can do* • Removed from home by adult protection because of concerns about night wandering and progressive dementia
Carol/son Andrew	83	Stonebridge	*This location works* • Moved from apartment after loss of husband, unable to care for self due to progressive dementia

6.5.2.2 Observations

Qualitative observations are those in which the researcher takes field notes on the behavior and activities of individuals at a particular research site. In these field notes, the researcher records in an unstructured or semi-structured way (Creswell, 2009). The goal of the observations in the two study facilities was to understand the physical and social interactions between residents, family caregivers, and care staff. An observation protocol was used to record the information in this research, with sections available for recording descriptions of the physical setting, accounts of a particular event or activity, description of particular participants, and reconstruction of dialogue (Creswell, 2009). In the Ridgemont community, these interactions took place in the memory care neighborhood public seating areas. In the Stonebridge

Theme	Definition	Example
Family Member	Discussion relating to the burden and transitions for family members when a resident is moved to LTC	
Caregiver Burden	Discussion relating to the burden of caring for a loved one with dementia at home	–And again, you're up all night, you have to work all day, and then you're up all night again; it's too much after a while
Transitions	Discussion relating to the circumstances surrounding the move of a family member to LTC	–He got out of their house and somebody found him at 5:30 in the morning at the side of the road, he had frost bite on his feet. They took him to the hospital, adult protection stepped in and two days later he was here. –One day my brother came home and Dad had built a fire in the middle of the living room because he said he was cold. Pretty soon after that he had to go to the hospital with pneumonia, that's when we sort of realized that he was not really able to handle the transition back home.
Anger and Guilt	Discussion relating to the emotions relating to the decision to move a family member into LTC	–I am still angry that this is happening and the lack of control. I feel guilty sometimes that I have done something wrong.
Letting Go	Discussion relating to the circumstances behind the resident's move and adjustment to LTC	–I'll get a phone call, which bothered me at first, but now I just listen and let him rant. –For the betterment of everybody, he is here. –

Fig. 6.2 Emergent themes

community, these interactions took place in the memory care household. Field notes were taken daily and included general impressions of observations and notation of the areas used by residents for public social activities.

6.5.3 Data Analysis

After the initial interviews were transcribed, the interviews and observational field notes were assessed, leading to a fracturing, or rearranging, of the data into categories which aided in the development of theoretical concepts. This coding or labeling was used to assign meaning to the data compiled (Miles & Huberman, 1994). Themes were analyzed for each of the two sites followed by a dissemination of interconnecting themes. The emergent themes for family caregivers were directly related to the transitions which had taken place through the continuum of care (Fig. 6.2). These themes included: (1) caregiver burden; (2) transitions; (3) anger and guilt; and (4) letting go.

6.6 Study Findings

6.6.1 Caregiver Burden

A constellation of factors are associated with stress resistance or resilience in dementia care, including contextual, care recipient status, and resource indicators (Gaugler, Pot, & Zarit, 2007). Rose and Bruce (1995) have described the emotions that go into caring for family members with dementia as a large part of the invisible work carried out by the caregiver. Levine et al. (2010) have written that, at the end of the day, for caregivers in demanding situations, there is no end of the day. Participants in the current study described the exhaustion and sleepless nights during the time their family member was living with them at home. Study participant John described the ups and downs in caring for his father George, now a Ridgemont resident, when he was still living at home: "When he was living with us, we would find things in his trash can that shouldn't be there, we'd find his socks in his water container. One day, he told us that someone one had stolen his glasses, and we told them that he was wearing them and he said, "Yeah, well I stole them back." While John and his wife were determined to keep his father at home, John recounts the point when the care became impossible due to his full time job, "At first Dad was sort of just rummaging, not really wandering, but rummaging. Things got worse and he was having a really hard time and would have hallucinations at night time, night terrors. I'd be up all night with him, then have to work all day, and then be up all night again, it's too much after a while."

Another Ridgemont family member, Joan, explains that her husband Tom's early life was defined by a very controlling father and then many subsequent years of his own alcoholism:

> Tom's been depressed all of his life. He has had these problems since he's been young, his parent divorced when he was 11. Nobody wanted him, so they shipped him off to a college. So he's had a difficult time, I wonder if that has to do with his dementia or not? And he drank, he was an alcoholic, he'd try and stop. We knew there was something wrong a while back when he used to go into rages that weren't typical of him.

Joan was concerned about these behaviors, yet when Tom would visit the doctor, he was able to get through the assessments for dementia by memorizing the questions. It was not until he was admitted to the hospital for pneumonia that he received a dementia diagnosis.

Other study participants experienced firsthand the unknowns and safety concerns that come with living with a someone with dementia. These safety concerns are not only for the care recipients, but the family members as well. For example, Ridgemont resident Frank began to show disruptive behaviors prior to moving to Ridgemont. His daughter Tina describes life with her father while he was living at home:

We tried to hire a home care helper, but Dad was extremely unable to deal with a stranger in the house, and would not recognize them or he would recognize them favorably for a half an hour and then would become extremely troubled and aggressive like, "Why is this person in my house?" It just wasn't working. Then he kind of got a bit like that with us too.

Frank had been fairly autonomous until he was stopped by a policeman for reckless driving and the officer decided to escort him home and took his driver's license away. For Tina, even without the use of the car, it seemed that her father had an inexhaustible supply of things that he could hurt himself or other people with. She said, "Dad is a real guy's guy; in his workbench he has every kind of knife, every kind of machine that could hurt you. One day my brother came home and Dad had built a fire in the middle of the living room because he said he was cold. In August, we started unplugging the stove and putting things up." Soon after that Frank was admitted to the hospital with pneumonia and the doctors finally made a diagnosis of dementia.

Stonebridge resident Vincent was in and out of the hospital several times in the year prior to his move to LTC. His wife Elizabeth explains that she had already come to an understanding that he needed to be in a LTC setting, due to many mini strokes and bowel cancer. She recalls how difficult the months were leading up to Vincent's move to Stonebridge, when he cycled in and out of the hospital due to his medical issues, "He found out about the cancer and dementia on the very same day, so it was two blows in 1 day. From September, which was the last time I brought him home from the hospital down home, from September to December, it was 24/7 care. I was just so exhausted."

Overall, respondents expressed their determination to keep their family member safe and comfortable, despite the challenges of the progression of the dementia illness and its impact on their own health. Many respondents were juggling work and family responsibilities during this period of time, and their caregiving role was an unquestioned added responsibility. It was not until an event left the caregiver with nowhere to turn but the DSW that discussions began about a permanent move to LTC.

6.6.2 *Transitions*

Commonly cited reasons for the decision for institutionalization include caregiver perceptions that dementia related problem behaviors are too difficult to handle (Buhr et al., 2006), yet the transition period from home or hospital to LTC can also be a stressful, trying time. The dynamics of the move can take its toll on both the care recipient and their family members, because a medical emergency often puts the family in shock mode rather than a planning mode (Roberts, 2012). Poorly planned and implemented transitions are prone to miscommunication, medication errors, and other lapses in patient safety. In turn, these lapses are costly and trauma of repeated cycles of transitions may lead to rapid deterioration and even death (Levine et al., 2010). How caregivers experience this trying time of waiting and transition is a vital area for exploration, particularly in the continuing care system in Nova Scotia designed to allow for smooth transitions for care recipients and their family members.

One of the principle elements of the single entry access system in Nova Scotia is that when there has been a determination of need for care, the individual is moved into the first available LTC bed in order to receive care until a bed becomes available in the community of choice. This process may, in itself, lead to stress for the family members and the resident may decompensate at an accelerated rate as they wait in a temporary situation for their desired location. This system allows for three chances to bypass the move in order to wait for a preferred facility, but if at the end of the third chance the individual has not moved, he or she goes back to the bottom of the list.

Exceptions are made, with variances that can get automatic placement in a care setting due to critical situations. That is when the move is from home, but due to back-ups in the hospitals, those waiting in the hospital will need to take the first available bed offered to them, waiting sometimes for days or weeks in transitional or acute care for a LTC bed to open. During this time, care levels may change, yet care needs reassessments do not take place until the transition to LTC has taken place. Joan explains how the bottlenecks in the healthcare system led to a series of break downs in resources available to her husband Tom:

> When Tom was able to come home from his stay in the hospital due to pneumonia, we waited for a home care assessment, but it took them four months to come and assess him. Then it took another six months until they called me and said they could give me an hour and a half of home health care in the morning. I said, "Well, you're a little late, he fell and broke his hip."

Tom spent several weeks in the hospital following hip surgery, and then was ready for transitional care. Transitional care in Nova Scotia is a sector of the hospital system where many frail older adults who have been in the hospital, but who no longer sick enough to be in acute care, are held until there is an open long term care bed. This is an "in-between" place, something of a "purgatory," where many patients may decompensate, both physically and cognitively, because of the lack of stimulation, and an undefined length of stay. Residents may be left to wait indefinitely in transitional care, sometimes at the end of that wait to be sent to the wrong community altogether.

At the time that Tom was waiting for a bed to open at Ridgemont, there were no available openings in transitional care, therefore he was kept in acute care for several months, while he waited for a bed to open in a nursing home. As Joan recalls, "They just kept him at the hospital, so they started charging him what the nursing home would charge. The whole thing was a nightmare and I'm not the only one that goes through it, it's the system but it shouldn't be that way. This is not the way that this system is designed to work."

Tina's father Frank had a little smoother transition after being admitted to the hospital with pneumonia the year before. "When Dad was in the hospital with pneumonia, that's when we sort of realized that he was not really able to handle the transition back home. The hospital admission processor told us that we could make him an urgent case because of his dementia diagnosis. They would give us the first opening, so that's how he got here."

Vincent's family had already placed him on a waiting list to move into a nearby LTC setting close to home, as he had been in and out of the hospital many times that year. Then, that winter, he left his home on foot in the middle of the night and somebody found him at 5:30 in the morning on the side of the road with frost bite on his feet. After a brief stay at his local hospital, adult protective services stepped in and Vincent was brought to Stonebridge in a matter of days. Elizabeth remembers the sense of relief when adult services stepped in, "For the betterment of everyone, he was moved here. We had already decided that it was getting close to time."

Carmen, another Stonebridge family member, had seen signs of dementia in her father Richard for some time and neighbors would often report seeing him driving down the wrong side of the road. He still had his driver license when he had an accident and was never able to return home. Carmen remembers the accident and months of rehab, "That day Dad was going for his regular cup of coffee, then three minutes later a guy comes to my brother's door and said, 'Bill, you've got to come; your dad's been in an accident.' He had hit a culvert at about 80 miles an hour and had broken his back and his neck. They got him into an ambulance and he spent five months in the hospital."

Richard's family had chosen to have him move to Ridgemont following his stay in the hospital, but as Carmen recalls, he had to spend several more months in the hospital until a long term care bed became available, "Dad waited another three months in the hospital for a nursing home bed. Then when he was supposed to move to Ridgmont, they sent him to Oakdale instead, which is another 50 minutes away. So they sent him to the wrong nursing home, the hospital did. Finally, they realized that they had sent the wrong person, and we got him here, that was about two years ago."

Despite the goals of the Continuing Care Strategy, study respondent input suggests that appropriate systems are not in place to help mitigate the confusion and uncertainty around the transition into LTC. Family members were consistently at the mercy of a system which in theory was put in to place to aid in smooth transitions and alleviate wait times. Instead, backups in the system often led to lengthy acute and transition care stays for care recipients, and higher levels of stress about the unknowns of the system for caregivers. As participant Gill noted about his wife Terry's transitions prior to moving to Stonebridge, "Having her in the hospital was bad enough…not knowing when she would be able to leave the hospital was even worse. She ended up sharing a room with three other people in transitional care for months."

6.6.3 Anger and Guilt

For caregivers of individuals with dementia, the role changes associated with caring do not end with placement in LTC (Bramble et al., 2009). Once a permanent move to LTC has been made, caregivers face new practical realities such as changes in the family's financial situations, frequent trips to the long-term care facility, reduced control over the care provided to their relative, and taking on new responsibilities such as coordinating and monitoring care (Schulz, Belle, Czaja, McGinnis, Stevens & Zhang, 2004). Unresolved problems between the caregiver and recipient, and conflict with family and friends over the LTC placement, may also contribute to the caregiver's post institutionalization stress (Gaugler, Pot, & Zarit, 2007). On a personal level, caregivers may continue to feel they have broken a promise or failed to live up to parental/spousal obligations (Shulz et al. 2004). This may result in a sense of obligation to remain involved in day-to-day care activities in the new facility (Bramble et al., 2009).

Family members in this study agreed that the burden of caring for a family member at home was matched by the trauma of going through the process of relocating a family member to LTC. They felt relief in being able to put the care of a loved one into the trusted hands of someone else and being able to move on with their life. There was relief, but anger and guilt as well, as the burden of caring for the relative at home was replaced with guilt at placing that spouse or parent in a care community. Joan described her feelings about moving Tom into LTC:

> I am still angry that this is happening and the lack of control. I feel guilty sometimes that I have done something wrong, especially when he calls me 10–12 times a day and says, "Well, you haven't been here to see me." And I say, "Well, I was there yesterday Tom." He doesn't remember, time doesn't mean anything to him.

Similarly, Gill receives the brunt of his spouse Terry's anger now that she is at Stonebridge, and while he has come to accept it as part of his role as her husband, it is still difficult. "If I'm late, she lets me know it. The other day I came in and she starts giving me hell and I didn't know what it was for, something that happened about 30 years ago. She just sits there all day and thinks of stuff, she has nothing else to do."

In general, study participants were torn in their decision to finally let go of their caregiving responsibilities, though were often relieved that DHW would be making the final decision about the care transition. John and his wife visited few his father George every day for the first few months that he was at Ridgemont, but slowly the visits became less frequent to once a month, as work and family responsibilities replaced trips to visit his father.

6.6.4 Letting Go

Once their relative is admitted into long term care, over time family caregivers often become care monitors and advocates (Levine et al., 2010), and may continue to hold responsibilities and in many case provide direct care (Keefe & Fancey, 2000). There are multiple patterns of adaptation as time since the move increases, and caregivers become more familiar with and engaged in their duties. During this period of time, there is an opportunity to build resilience and coping strategies in order to manage care demands and other stressors (Gaugler, Pot, & Zarit, 2007), and relationships formed between care staff and well informed family members may also improve dementia care and service delivery once the transition in to LTC has taken place (Bramble et al., 2009).

Despite a 120 km drive, Vincent's wife Elizabeth continues to visit her husband at Stonebridge as frequently as she can. While she has been offered by the DHW to have Vincent transferred to another facility closer to home, she feels it's best not to move him again. She explains that she able to spend quality time with him now when she visits, "We sit and talk and if he's sleeping or cat napping, I just let him sleep. Sometimes when we want to eat together, I'll bring something in or have coffee or something. Other times we'll just walk around and chit chat, he and I have great conversations."

Elizabeth and her family feel that Vincent is well taken care of at Stonebridge. She explains that based on her income, the monthly cost for Vincent's care at Stonebridge is $1100. "He gets the care that he needs, and the cost is minimal, compared to what you'd face trying to do this on you own at home. The staff are extremely caring; they do what they can with that they have."

Another Stonebridge family member, Andrew, and five of his siblings trade off visiting his mother Carol and feel that the Stonebridge location works because it is so close to her old apartment, "Yes, she's comfortable, she likes it. We can take her out and she recognizes the neighborhood. The biggest problems are later in the evening with sundowners, but other than that, she likes it here, this location works." Andrew also sees that the frequent visits from family members have allowed important relationships to form with the care staff, "I think that if the family helps out a little bit it makes it better, much better. You also get to know the staff; you get to know them on a first name basis. I think that's really important."

A Ridgemont spouse, Garney, has visited his wife Rose every day. Not a just short visit, he comes in around 9 am and leaves around 4 pm, "Unless, of course, there's a snow storm or I'm sick." He is a fixture there, he knows all of the residents and staff by first name, and most days, sits next to Rose in her wheelchair and holds her hand whether she is asleep or awake. He is aware that she no longer recognizes him as her husband, yet is comfortable in his role, "I know that she knows that I am someone who cares about her." When asked if there is a time which he thinks he would move to Ridgemont too, in order to be with Rose full time, Garney is pragmatic and quick to answer, "We still have our home, someone needs to take care of it. I can do that, watch the ships in the Bedford Basin in the morning and be here to see Rose when she wakes up in the morning. Things are fine just as they are."

While these are not happy stories, the caregivers in this study have demonstrated the ability to let go a little bit. Joan will continue to visit Tom, at the same time moving on with her life as a mother and grandmother while her husband of 50-plus years continues his slide into the depths of a place where she can no longer reach him. Garney will keep the home that he and his wife Rose shared for almost five decades, while at the same time spending every day with her at Ridgemont. For Vincent's wife, children, and grandchildren who drive an hour each way to visit him, the peace of mind in knowing that he is being well-cared for in a safe environment affords them a sense of closure in knowing that they will not need to move him again.

6.7 Implications

6.7.1 Implications for Understanding Family Resilience

Transitions between care settings—in which family members play an important role—bring the varied elements of health and long-term care together for fleeting but critical moments in time. Therefore, the contributions and experiences of family caregivers through the trajectory of care should be considered in gathering information to shape policies and practice, training health care professionals, developing programs, and reforming financing (Levine et al., 2010).

The ability of some caregivers to persevere through these transitions may be due to multiple factors, including self-efficacy, familial support systems, health status of the care recipient and caregiver, and secondary community based services resulting in caregiver resilience (Gaugler, Pot, & Zarit, 2007). While the psychological conceptualization of resilience is the ability to maintain normal or enhanced functioning during times of adversity (Cherry et al., 2013), an individual's ability to transition to a new and similarly complex set of challenges through the continuum of care may test this resilience. Despite resolve and commitment to their caregiving role, without appropriate supports in place at each of these points of transition, the ability of the caregiver to remain resilient over time can be tested.

The voices of the family caregivers in this study reflect this, through their experiences at caregiving at home as well as through the continuing care system in their province. Respondents spoke of their fatigue in their caregiving role and the unknowns and safety concerns of the disease while their family member was still at home. While they were grateful for their DHW healthcare safety net, once there has been a decision to place a family member into a care setting outside of home, there are often the added factors of assessments and wait times to get into a long term care community. Respondents report that provincial DHW assessment policies often led to protracted transitions and extra time spent in the hospital or transitional care, creating more stress, as the individuals with dementia and the family members waited in limbo for a bed to open in a nursing community. Finally, letting go of the caregiving responsibility once a final move to LTC had taken place created a new, complex set of circumstances for the respondents. While some were able to settle into the rhythm of the care facility as an integral part of their family members' day, others had more difficulty, particularly when their family member had moved far enough into the disease where they no longer were able to communicate, leading to anger and guilt on the part of the caregiver.

The interviewees in this study have informed us that because dementia is a chronic, long term, and progressive disease, the needs for supportive services and programs will change over time. Therefore, rather than of an "on/off" conceptual-

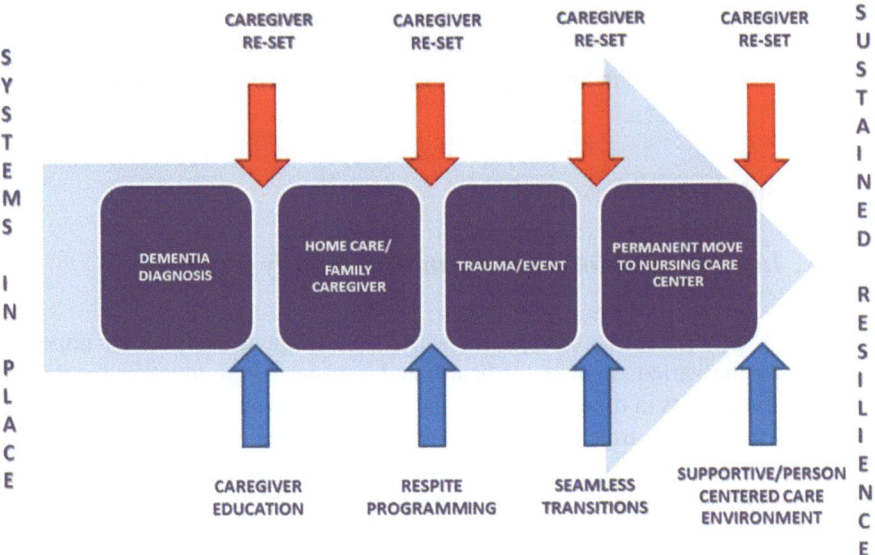

Fig. 6.3 Caregiver resilience through systems in place

ization of resilience, the focus instead should be the continuum of support both for the care giver and care recipient throughout the course of the dementia, because each care transition leads to a new set of concerns about the unknowns of the new phase for the family member (Fig. 6.3).

Developing models for supportive services in order to help caregivers maintain sustained resilience from the point of the dementia diagnosis *through* the point of a permanent placement in a LTC setting may not only be appropriate, but necessary, as the numbers of informal family caregivers continue to grow with an aging population. This will involve recognition by policy makers of caregivers as full partners in all aspects of the care provided, education of clinicians regarding the continuing role of the caregiver in the life of the resident with dementia after placement in LTC, and allowing family members to be integral in decision making regarding the direction of the care being provided (Strang et al., 2006). More time and money are important incentives to support care coordination, but new models and staff training are critical as well (Levine et al., 2010).

6.7.2 Implications for Practice and Policy

While families are the bedrock of long-term care, policy makers have traditionally considered them "informal" caregivers, as they are not part of the formal paid caregiving workforce. Yet as chronic and long-term care systems become more complex, and as more demanding tasks are shifted to families, this view is no longer sustainable. Policy makers are beginning to take the position that caregivers support must enhance involvement and training in order to contribute to reducing unnecessary rehospitalizations and improved patient outcomes (Levine et al., 2010). While the DHW in Nova Scotia took initial steps to mitigate the burden of care for family caregivers through the continuing care strategy, more work will need to be done to prepare caregivers for the trajectory of the disease and to allow for smoother transitions once a move is determined to be necessary.

It is hoped that the caregiver stories in this study may inform policy makers of the importance of support programs and services which take into consideration the changing needs of both the individual with dementia and the caregiver throughout the continuum of care. Creating assessment tools that identify resilient caregivers by means of their adaptation to stressful aspects of dementia caregiving situations may aid in targeting best practices in interventions and may help to delay or prevent key care transitions such as nursing home placement, as well as future health care needs of the family caregivers after they have relinquished their home caregiving responsibilities. In addition, community support systems should strive to offer support to caregivers to help diffuse some of the negative feelings of guilt, thus facilitating outcomes that are more positive for both caregiver and care recipient (Buhr et al., 2006).

At the time of this publication, Nova Scotia is moving toward a new provincial Dementia Strategy to create a common set of values and guiding principles for an integrated and coordinated support system for individuals with dementia and their families. Future studies will be critical in determining if the new strategy will address the needs of the stakeholders in a holistic way, providing support through the caregiving journey in order to aid in sustained resilience. Outcomes of this current study and future research have implications not only for the stakeholders in Nova Scotia and the other Canadian provinces, but for the current health care system in the United States, as well. U.S. policy makers continue to grapple with the relations between state and federal funding for dementia care and how to create a solid support system for an ever-growing population of individuals with dementia and the family members who care for them. Future policy should address the provision of a comprehensive continuing care system, so that caregivers can return to the important role of just being a husband, wife, son, or daughter, while at the same time negotiating their care journey with the necessary support systems in place.

Questions for Thought and Discussion

1. Discuss the confluence of feelings and responsibilities that family caregiving of individuals with dementia experience.
2. Using Fig. 6.1 and Fig. 6.3, describe the impact of supportive programming for caregiver resilience. Compare and contrast the two diagrams and how they relate to resilience for caregiver across the trajectory of care.
3. What are the similarities and differences between the Nova Scotia provincial Continuing Care Strategy for families caring for a family member with dementia and current U.S. policy and programming? What are some of the gaps in support

for family members in the Continuing Care Strategy and how might the strategy be improved?
4. Describe what is meant by the phase "anger and guilt, the one-two punch" with respect of family caregiving for individuals with dementia.
5. How would a caregiver's resilience be tested once a family member has been moved into a long-term care setting? What are some strategies that the caregiver might use to maintain their resilience once this transition has been made?

References

Abby, J., Froggard, K., Parker, D., & Abby, B. (2005). Palliative care in long term care: A system change. *Journal of Older People Nursing, 1,* 56–63. doi:10.1111/j.1748-3743.2006.00010.x

Alzheimer's Association. (2015). 2015 Alzheimer's disease facts and figures: Statistical resource for data related to Alzheimer's disease. *Alzheimer's & Dementia, 11,* 332–384. doi:10.1016/j.jalz.2015.02.003

Banerjee, A. (2009). Long-term care in Canada: An overview. In P. Armstrong (Ed.), *A place to call home: Long term care in Canada.* Nova Scotia, CA: Fernwood.

Bramble, M., Moyle, W., & McAllister, M. (2009). Seeking connection: Family care experiences following long-term dementia care placement. *Journal of Clinical Nursing, 18,* 3118–3125. doi:10.1111/j.1365-2702.2009.02878.x

Brodaty, H., & Donkin, M. (2009). Family caregivers of people with dementia. *Dialogues in Clinical Neuroscience, 11,* 217–228.

Buhr, G., Kuchibhatla, M., & Clipp, E. (2006). Caregivers' reasons for nursing home placement: Clues for improving discussions with families prior to the transition. *The Gerontologist, 46,* 52–61. doi:10.1093/geront/46.1.52

Caron, C. D., & Bowers, B. J. (2003). Deciding whether to continue, share, or relinquish caregiving: Caregiver views. *Qualitative Health Research, 13*(9), 1252–1271. doi:10.1177/1049732303257236

Caron, C. D., Ducharme, F., & Griffith, J. (2006). Deciding on institutionalization for a relative with dementia: The most difficult decision for caregivers. *Canadian Journal on Aging, 25*(2), 193–205.

Chaudhury, H. (2002). Journey back home. *Journal of Housing for the Elderly, 16*(1–2), 85–106. doi:10.1300/J081v16n01_07

Cherry, M. G., Salmon, P., Dickson, J. M., Powell, D., Sikdar, S., & Ablett, J. (2013). Factors influencing resilience of carers of individuals with dementia. *Reviews in Clinical Gerontology, 23,* 251–266. doi:10.1017/S0959259813000130

Connidis, I. A. (2010). *Family ties and aging.* Los Angeles, CA: Pine Forge Press.

Creswell, J. (2009). *Research design: Qualitative, quantitative and mixed method approaches.* Los Angeles, CA: Sage.

Feinberg, L. F., Newman, S. L., Gray, L., & Kolb, K. N. (2004). *The state of the states in family caregiver support: A 50-state study.* San Francisco, CA: Family Caregiver Alliance.

Gaugler, J. E., Kane, R. L., & Newcomer, R. (2007). Resilience and transitions from dementia caregiving. *Journal of Gerontology: Psychological Sciences, 62B,* 38–44. doi:10.1093/geronb/62.1.P38

Gaugler, J. E., Leach, C. R., Clay, T., & Newcomer, R. C. (2004). Predictors of nursing home placement in African Americans with dementia. *Journal of the American Geriatrics Society, 52,* 445–452. doi:10.1111/j.1532-5415.2004.52120.x

Gaugler, J. E., Pot, A. M., & Zarit, S. (2007). Long-term adaptation to institutionalization in dementia caregivers. *The Gerontologist, 47,* 730–740. doi:10.1093/geront/47.6.730

Geda, Y., Schneider, L., Gitlin, L., Miller, D., Smith, G., Bell, J., ... Lyketsos, C. (2013). Neuropsychiatric symptoms of Alzheimer's disease: Past progress and anticipation of the future. *Alzheimer's & Dementia*, *9*, 602–608. doi:10.1016/j.jalz.2012.12.001

Guberman, N. (2005). *Assessment of family caregivers: A practice perspective*. Prepared for National Consensus Development Conference for Caregiver Assessment. San Francisco, CA: Family Caregiver Alliance.

Keefe, J., & Fancey, P. (2000). The care continues: Responsibility for elderly relatives before and after admission to a long term care facility. *Family Relations*, *19*, 235–244. doi:10.1111/j.1741-3729.2000.00235.x

Levine, C., Halper, D., Peist, A., & Gould, D. (2010). Bridging troubled waters: Family caregivers, transitions, and long-term care. *Health Affairs*, *29*, 116–124. doi:10.1377/hlthaff.2009.0520

Maas, M., Reed, D., Park, M., Specht, J., Schutte, D., Kelley, I., ... Buckwalter, K. (2004). Outcomes of family involvement in care: Intervention for caregivers of individuals with dementia. *Nursing Research*, *53*, 76–78. doi:10.1097/00006199-200403000-00003

Miles, M. B., & Huberman, A. M. (1994). *Qualitative data analysis*. Thousand Oaks, CA: Sage. doi:10.1016/0022-3999(96)00056-6

Nova Scotia Department of Health and Wellness. (2006). *Shaping the future of continuing care in Nova Scotia: To have every Nova Scotian live in a place they can call home*. Report from the Provincial Steering Committee.

Nova Scotia Department of Health and Wellness. (2015). *Towards understanding: A dementia strategy for Nova Scotia* (pp. 1–35). Province of Nova Scotia, CA: Dept. of Health and Wellness.

Park, M., Butcher, H. K., & Mass, M. L. (2004). The thematic analysis of Korean family caregivers' experiences in making the decision to place a family member with dementia in a long term care facility. *Research in Nursing and Health*, *27*, 345–356. doi:10.1002/nur.20031

Raina, P., O'Donnell, M., Schwellnus, H., Rosenbaum, P., King, G., Brehaut, J., ... Wood, E. (2004). Caregiving process and caregiver burden: Conceptual models to guide research and practice. *BMC Pediatrics*, *4*, 1–13. doi:10.1186/1471-2431-4-1

Roberts, E. (2012). *Legislating home: The impact of the regulation of small house settings for long term care residents in Nova Scotia, CA*. (Unpublished doctoral dissertation). University of Missouri-Columbia.

Rose, H., & Bruce, H. (1995). Mutual care but differential esteem: Caring between older couples. In S. Arber & J. Ginn (Eds.), *Connecting gender and aging: A sociological approach* (pp. 114–128). Buckingham, UK: Open University Press.

Ross, L., Holliman, D., & Dixon, D. R. (2003). Resiliency in family caregivers: Implications for social work practice. *Journal of Gerontological Social Work*, *40*, 81–96. doi:10.1300/J083v40n03_07

Rubenstein, R. L. (2002). The qualitative interview with older informants: Some key questions. In G. Rowles & N. Schoenberg (Eds.), *Qualitative gerontology: A contemporary perspective*. New York, NY: Springer.

Schulz, R., Belle, S. H., Czaia, S. J., McGinnis, K. A., Stevens, A., & Zhang, S. (2004). Long-term care placement of dementia patients and caregiver health and well-being. *Journal of the American Medical Association*, *292*(8), 961–967.

Strang, V., Koop, P., Dupuis-Blanchard, S., Nordstrom, M., & Thompson, B. (2006). Family caregivers and transition to long-term care. *Clinical Nursing Research*, *15*, 27–45. doi:10.1177/1054773805282356

Walsh, F. (2003). Family resilience: A framework for clinical practice. *Family Process*, *42*, 1–18. doi:10.1111/j.1545-5300.2003.00001.x

Chapter 7
Planning for and Managing Costs Related to Caregiving

Louise A. Schroeder and Sissy R. Osteen

"Will my money last as long as I do?" "Will I outlive my money?" These are common questions asked by retirees. An article titled "How to Make Your Money Last" by Jane Bryant Quinn in the January–February, 2016 issue of the AARP Bulletin addresses these questions (Quinn, 2016). It includes a discussion of types of retirement plans to use for accumulating for retirement, strategies for withdrawing money during retirement, and retirement mistakes to avoid. All of this is good information, but there isn't any discussion of how caregiving, either needing it or providing it, can impact retirement income and assets.

Anyone who has ever been, or is now, a caregiver can attest to the reality that caregiving is different for each care recipient. Some caregivers might choose to think of the experience as an adversity, others think of it as a challenge, and still others think of it as a privilege. Regardless of the perspectives of the caregiver and the care recipient, caregiving always involves time, effort, and money. The potential for costs to be devastating to the care recipient, the unpaid caregiver(s), or both is well-documented and of great concern. An Issue Brief from the Office of the Assistant Secretary for Planning and Evaluation (ASPE), Office of Disability, Aging and Long-Term Care Policy (Favrealt & Dey, 2015) states that for some, the costs of long-term services and support (long-term care) are likely to outstrip retirement savings. Also, an Issue Brief from the Employee Benefit Research Institute (VanDerHei, 2015) states that nursing home and home health care costs can have catastrophic financial consequences for the future retirement income adequacy of the household. Developing and implementing a financial plan before something

---

L.A. Schroeder, CFP® (✉)
Certified Financial Planner™ Professional, PO Box 1267, Stillwater, OK 74076, USA
e-mail: louise@louiseschroeder.net

S.R. Osteen, Ph.D., CFP®
Human Development and Family Science, Oklahoma State University, Stillwater, OK 74074, USA
e-mail: sissy.osteen@okstate.edu

happens can provide a sense of security, and can ease the stress of managing the financial impact of caregiving.

Helping families and individuals plan financially for the possible need for caregiving for themselves, for family members, or for friends (at any age) is challenging because this has not been a well-defined area of financial planning. For the same reason, the management of costs that occur during a period of caregiving are just as challenging. A large number of the articles related to the post-retirement period of life that have appeared in financial planning professional journals and publications have, for the most part, covered topics related to accumulating assets for retirement, strategies for structuring income flows during retirement, investment strategies for retirement assets, long-term care decisions (focused on the need for skilled care), and estate planning.

There is a need for synthesizing information from the field of gerontology with information from the field of financial planning/management in order to expand and better define the area of financial planning addressing the financial issues of older adults, and caregiving in particular. Since the reader may not have a clear idea of what financial planning encompasses, a discussion of basic financial planning concepts is provided. This is followed by a discussion of the aging environment from the perspective of information that is pertinent to the data gathering portion of the financial planning process. Understanding the aging environment and what caregiving encompasses will help the financial planner to do a better job of analyzing and evaluating the individual's or family's financial situation, which is necessary in order to make good recommendations.

7.1 Financial Planning Concepts

What is financial planning? If that question is "googled" on web browsers such as Mozilla Foxfire or Chrome, what appears first on the computer screen are ads placed by firms that sell financial products such as investments, insurance, and annuities. A website link that may appear near the top of the list of related websites is for Investopedia (Investopedia, 2016, January), which states the following: "Definition of Financial Plan: A comprehensive evaluation of an investor's current and future financial state by using currently known variables to predict future cash flows, asset values and withdrawal plans." A common perception is that financial planning focuses on investment advising (note the use of the word investor in this definition). Financial planning encompasses a great deal more than just investing advice.

A more complete definition can be found on the Certified Financial Planner Board of Standards website (CFP Board of Standards, 2016, January). The CFP Board of Standards defines financial planning as the process of determining whether and how an individual can meet life goals through the proper management of financial resources. Financial planning integrates the financial planning process with the financial planning subject areas.

Six steps are listed on the website for the financial planning process:
1. Establishing and defining the client-planner relationship
2. Gathering client data including goals
3. Analyzing and evaluating the client's current financial status
4. Developing and presenting recommendations and/or alternatives
5. Implementing the recommendations
6. Monitoring the recommendations

The website states that the phrase "financial planning subject areas" denotes the basic subject fields covered in the financial planning process which typically include, but are not limited to:

Financial statement preparation and analysis (including cash flow analysis/planning and budgeting)
Insurance planning and risk management
Employee benefits planning
Investment planning
Income tax planning
Retirement planning
Estate planning

So, where does planning for caregiving fit in? Because of the potentially devastating financial impact, risk management is a common choice because it most frequently deals with the use of insurance in mitigating a variety of potentially devastating financial risks. Three types of insurance, medical (Medicare/Medicaid for those 65+), disability, and long-term care, are useful in the caregiving environment. However, while they will pay for specific types of expenses, they have limited or no application in addressing many of the wide variety of direct and indirect costs related to caregiving.

Financial planning for caregiving encompasses parts of each of the subject areas listed above, but it also requires information about, knowledge of, and an understanding of concepts that are not included in any of these areas. Development of a knowledge base that includes information from the field of gerontology will enable financial planners to work more effectively with families, individuals, and professionals who work in the caregiving field. More effective planning for potential caregiving expenses and management of those expenses during the caregiving period, if and when it occurs, will contribute to family and individual resilience.

The concept of fiduciary duty is currently a frequent topic of discussion in the financial industry. Exactly what fiduciary duty means has not yet been clarified. There is a general sense that it includes putting a client's best interest first; this is referred to as a duty of loyalty. A duty of care has also been part of the discussion and this has been defined, in part, as being competent to give financial advice. This underscores the importance of understanding the aging environment and factors that can impact caregiving decisions in order to provide more effective planning.

7.2 The Goal of Successful Aging

A goal that is commonly expressed by individuals when planning their retirement years is to age successfully. How each individual defines the concept of successful aging can vary widely. What constitutes successful aging has been the subject for a number of research projects. A comprehensive, inter-disciplinary research project conducted by the MacArthur Foundation starting in 1984 resulted in a book published in 1998 (Rowe & Kahn, 1998). The authors define successful aging as effective functioning in later life, and further as "the ability to maintain three key behaviors or characteristics: low risk of disease and disease-related

> **Breakout Box 7.1 Focus on Practice**
> **When do people think about planning for the possibility of becoming a caregiver or needing caregiving themselves?**
> As a Certified Financial Planner™ professional with a private practice, I am getting more and more questions from clients about caregiving topics. Some of the questions relate to planning for their own later years of life. These questions focus on when to start this kind of planning, where to live in the later years of their lives, whether or not they should purchase long-term care insurance, how to decide about who should care for them, what kind of help may be needed and how to find it, etc. These questions often come when they are either getting close to retiring or have already retired and they need to make decisions related to what they want for this period of their lives. Sometimes questions come up when they are involved in doing estate planning. More infrequently questions may arise when clients are looking at disability insurance and beginning to think about "what if..." situations.
>
> The majority of questions are concerning issues their own parents are facing and how to best help their parents. Often they are dealing with these issues because of an "event" such as an illness or injury or the death of one of their parents, or realizing that their parents are needing help more often and they want to work with family members to meet the needs of their aging parents. Also, I have had to start giving thought to how I can work with clients who are living with cognitive impairment issues and their families and friends who are their unpaid caregivers.
>
> This is an area of financial planning that I did not receive training in when I studied to obtain my CFP® designation. Thankfully, more attention is being given to topics related to helping clients who are unpaid caregivers, as well as clients who are becoming more interested in planning for the time when they may need care. Clients do not want to burden their own families and friends, and understand that planning ahead gives everyone more comfort.

disability; high mental and physical functioning; and active engagement with life" (p. 38).

Another study, the National Institute on Aging's Baltimore Longitudinal Study of Aging, was started in 1958 to provide answers to the question: What is normal aging? (Hodes, Longo, & Ferrucci, 2010). Two conclusions based on this research are that normal aging is separate from disease and there is not just one chronological timetable of human aging. In his book about planning for retirement years, Certified Financial Planner™ professional Michael Stein includes nine factors as influencing a prosperous retirement: (1) finances, (2) physical health, (3) mental health, (4) diet, (5) exercise, (6) social relations, (7) personal relations, (8) intellectual stimulation, and (9) spiritual balance (Stein, 1998).

Caregiving can easily over-shadow the other aspects of a care recipient's life even though they remain important to the care recipient. The financial planning process includes defining the individual's goals for his or her life, so caregiving goals would be integrated with goals that are important to the individual in the other areas. Allocating financial resources (income and assets) for caregiving can easily cause goals in other areas to be overlooked.

7.3 Understanding the Aging Environment

Step two of the financial planning process focuses on gathering data. This generally involves a questionnaire that asks for personal information, financial information, and the individual's or couple's goals. It also includes an in depth discussion of the information revealed in the questionnaire. Knowing what questions to ask in order to obtain the appropriate information needed to complete the rest of the financial planning process is imperative. Certainly, understanding issues associated with the aging population (both within the U. S. and worldwide), is helpful in developing questions related to planning for caregiving.

While it is common knowledge that members of the baby boom generation have been reaching the age of 65 at a rate of 10,000 per day since January 2011, and will continue to do so through the end of 2029, understanding the significance of this demographic shift to an older population is critical. A report issued by the Stanford Center on Longevity provides a framework for thinking about critical trends associated with an older America (Hayutin, Dietz, & Mitchell, 2010).

The report focuses on important changes in the following areas:
- Population aging
- Increased racial and ethnic diversity
- Changes in living arrangements
- Evolving health care needs
- Challenges to financial well-being

7.3.1 Population Aging

The Administration on Aging, Administration for Community Living, and the U.S. Department of Health and Human Services annually issue a report with statistics on the older population (Administration on Aging, 2014). The report states that the population aged 65 and over was at 44.7 million in 2013 and will almost double to 82.3 million by 2040. Of that 44.7 million people, 25.1 million are female and 19.6 million are male. The population aged 85 and over is expected to almost triple from 6 million in 2013 to 14.6 million in 2040. The number of Americans age 100+ rose 45% from 2000 to 2014. Not only is the 65+ population growing in size and as a percentage of the total population, they are living much longer. This means that they are more likely to live to an age when caregiving may be needed. This will have a long-term impact on the demand for caregiving services, and for more care providers (both paid and unpaid). Increasing numbers of older adults also suggests that the potential for more adults ages 45–64 to be involved with caregiving will also increase. These adult children are predominantly unpaid caregivers who are working and are impacted in a number of ways themselves, which are discussed in Sect. 7.5.3.

Marital demographic statistics change as people age. In 2014, 72% of males 65+ were married compared to 46% of females. Older adult women were more likely to be widowed than men, 35% versus 11%. The percentage of divorced/separated older persons increased to 14.1% in 2014 from 5.3% in 1980 (Administration on Aging, 2014). These statistics will continue to change as the population ages, and indicate that older women are more likely to be cared for by family members or paid care providers, than by spouses.

7.3.2 Increased Racial and Ethnic Diversity

By 2042 more than half the population will be non-white or Hispanic. The U.S. population is expected to grow from 310 million in 2010 to 439 million in 2050. The white non-hispanic population is projected to only grow from 201 million in 2010 to 203 million in 2050. The number of Hispanics is forecast to grow from 50 million in 2010 to 133 million in 2050, which makes it the fastest growing population segment. The African American population is expected to grow from 38 million in 2010 to 52 million in 2050. It is important to note that racial and ethnic groups differ on life expectancy, living arrangements, disease prevalence, income levels, and poverty rates (Hayutin et al., 2010). These factors will add complexity to the concept of caregiving and to what the reality of caregiving will be for caregivers in each of these segments of the population. Financial planners will need to understand cultural differences among these segments of the population in order to provide recommendations that are in the individual's and the family's best interests.

7.3.3 Change in Living Arrangements

Where is the older population living now and where will they be living in the future? Will they choose to remain in the single family homes where they raised their children and have continued to live in retirement? Will they choose to downsize to houses that are smaller in size and that require less maintenance? Will they move to independent living senior neighborhoods designed for the 55+ market? Will they opt for a continuing care retirement community that offers independent living, assisted living, and/or skilled care/memory care units where they can move from one area to another if and when the need arises? Will they stay in their own homes until a move to assisted living or skilled care or memory care housing is required? The options that are currently available are many, and new housing options will continue to be developed to meet the needs of our aging population. Where caregiving takes place can make a considerable difference in the costs related to caregiving.

A report published by the Center for Housing Policy, which is the research division of the non-profit National Housing Conference, indicates that based on information from the 2009 American Housing Survey 23% of U.S. households included someone age 65 and older. In 12% of households the oldest member was 65–74, in 8% the oldest member was 75–84, and in 3% the oldest member was 85+. Statistics in 2011 indicated that of 13 million households with the oldest member being 65–74, 18% were renting, 32% owned the house and had a mortgage, and 50% owned the house with the mortgage paid off. Of 9.1 million households with the oldest member being 75–84, the percentages were 20%, 19%, and 62%. Of 3.8 million households with the oldest member being 85+, the percentages were 24%, 16%, and 61%. This report also indicates that while 6% of adults age 65+ live in physically inadequate conditions, many housing units may be neither safe nor suitable for older adults (Lipman, Lubell, & Salomon, 2012). Modifying existing housing to make the houses both safe and functional for older adults can become expensive. There is a need for building houses that are designed for life-long living, and this can be done at less expense than modifying existing houses.

Another report from the Joint Center for Housing Studies of Harvard University states that the majority of the 50+ population live independently within the community versus in institutional care facilities (Joint Center for Housing Studies of Harvard University, 2014). A 2010 Census Bureau special studies report on the 65+ population provides more detail about where people live by age group. Of the 65–74 age group, 98% live in a traditional community, while 1% live in community housing with services (retirement community, continuing care retirement community, assisted living facility), and the remaining 1% live in a long-term care facility. For the age group 74–84 the percentages are 93%, 3%, and 4%, and for the 85+ group they are 78%, 7%, and 15% (West, Cole, Goodkind, & He, 2010).

Of particular concern when caregiving is needed is whether the individual lives alone, with a spouse, or with a family member or someone else. The 2010 Census Bureau report provides information about those who live alone by age and sex. In the 65–74 age group, 15.6% of males live alone versus 26.4% of females. In the 75–84 age group, 19.1% of males live alone while 39% of females do. In the 85–94 age group, 27% of males live alone, while 47.6% of females do. In the 95+ age group 33.4% of males live alone, while 36.8% of females do (West et al., 2014).

An AARP research report states that the desire to age in place was indicated by 90% of adults age 65+, and that 80% believe their current residence is where they will always live (Farber, Shinkle, Lynott, Fox-Grage, & Harrell, 2011). A report published by the Bipartisan Policy Center Housing Commission defines aging in place as the ability to live in one's own home and community safely, independently, and comfortably, regardless of age, income, or ability level. It also states that for most seniors, the desire to age at home is the most cost-effective and financially sensible housing option, as long as they are physically able. Yet, the reality of homes and neighborhoods that were designed before current demographic trends began to shift can present a number of barriers for many seniors and elders. It further states that the homes of many seniors lack the necessary structural features and support systems that can make independent living into old age a viable, safe option (Housing Commission, 2013). These concerns must be considered when decisions are being weighed as to where may be the best place to live for a person who needs assistance. The costs for updating an existing home must be compared to the costs related to other types of living options.

The federal government has also recognized that aging in their own homes in the communities where they live is more cost effective for older adults, as well as for the federal and state governments, and results in a better quality of life for those older adults receiving benefits. A significant example of this comes from a report issued by the Centers for Medicare and Medicaid Services and the Department of Health and Human Services (Centers for Medicare and Medicaid Services, 2017). Under the section on Providing Long Term Services and Supports in the Community it states that Medicaid provides half of the nation's long-term care. Also, that in 2013 for the first time the majority (52%) of Medicaid spending on long-term services and supports was for home and community based services rather than for institutional care, and that this continues to increase.

7.3.4 Evolving Health Care Needs

Very few individuals age 65+ avoid having at least one of many health conditions that affect their quality of life, and that impact their need for caregiving. The Baltimore Longitudinal Study of Aging found that while normal aging is not directly related to disease, the two are not independent of each other either. One of the BLSA's current areas of research, the Insight into the Determinants of Exceptional Aging and Longevity (IDEAL), focuses on people 80 years and older who are living free of physical and cognitive disease. The goal of this study is to identify factors that distinguish extraordinary health at very advanced ages from non-ideal aging (Hodes et al., 2010).

A 2010 report on chronic health conditions from the Department of Health and Human Services defines chronic illnesses as conditions that last a year or more and require ongoing medical attention and/or limit activities of daily living (DHHS, 2010). In 2011, approximately 67.3% of Medicare beneficiaries had two or more chronic conditions and 14% had six or more. That 14% of beneficiaries accounted for almost half of total Medicare spending. The Centers for Medicare and Medicaid Services Chronic Conditions Warehouse database tracks information on pre-defined indicators for the following chronic conditions: Alzheimer's/related dementias, arthritis, asthma, atrial fibrillation, cancer (breast, colorectal, lung, & prostate), chronic kidney disease, chronic obstructive pulmonary disease, depression, diabetes, heart failure, hyperlipidemia, hypertension, ischemic heart disease, osteoporosis, and stroke (Centers for Medicare and Medicaid Services, 2014).

The prevalence of multiple chronic conditions among Medicare beneficiaries in 2011 was:

Medicare beneficiaries with 0–1 chronic conditions ~32.7%
Medicare beneficiaries with 2–3 chronic conditions ~31.5%
Medicare beneficiaries with 4–5 chronic conditions ~21.8%
Medicare beneficiaries with 6+ chronic conditions ~14.0%

Statistics related to how much Medicare spends per beneficiary based on their number of chronic conditions are sobering:

Medicare spending for beneficiaries with 0–1 chronic conditions = $2,097
Medicare spending for beneficiaries with 2–3 chronic conditions = $5,677
Medicare spending for beneficiaries with 4–5 chronic conditions = $11,628
Medicare spending for beneficiaries with 6+ chronic conditions = $31,543

For Oklahoma Medicare beneficiaries the figures were $2,038, $5,971, $12,512, and $32,073 (Lochner, Goodman, Posner, & Parekh, 2013).

While these figures represent expenses paid by Medicare, each individual also incurs expenses. Each individual pays a premium for Medicare Part B and Part D or Medicare Part C (some individuals pay a surcharge based on their income); deductibles for Medicare Part A, Part B, and Part D or Part C (the deductible for Part A can be charged more than once per calendar year, and there are no out-of-pocket limits per individual for Part A); Medicare co-insurance/copays for Parts A, B, and D or Part C; a premium for Medicare Supplemental insurance (by choice, this is not mandatory); costs of lab tests and diagnostic procedures, etc. that exceed Medicare limits on frequency; and health care costs not covered by Medicare. Many costs related to caregiving are not covered by Medicare (Centers for Medicare and Medicaid Services, 2016).

Having multiple chronic conditions is an indicator that an individual is more likely to need assistance with activities of daily living such as eating, bathing, dressing, mobility, transferring, toileting, and incontinence. Initially these individuals may need help with instrumental activities of daily living such as home maintenance (inside and outside), yard maintenance, meal preparation, shopping, transportation, managing money/investments/legal issues, making appointments, communicating with professionals, using a telephone or computer, taking medications, and more. The inability to perform many of these activities can severely restrict an individual's quality of life (Centers for Disease Control and Prevention, 2013). Assistance with these types of activities is not covered by Medicare and is most often provided by unpaid, informal caregivers.

Taking into consideration the demographic information presented earlier, especially the fact that the U.S. (and worldwide) population age 65+ is increasing at a faster rate than younger segments of the population and that people age 65+ are living longer, the impacts are far reaching. Such impacts will be felt by federal, state, and local government agencies and programs, businesses/employers, organizations, non-profits, and family members/friends will be tremendous and impact families of all backgrounds and types. This makes planning for the potential of needing caregiving or having to provide caregiving critical. For the most part, individuals wait until an event such as a sudden injury, an unexpected illness, or the death of a spouse/partner occurs, and then decisions are made more on a reactionary basis versus an informed basis.

7.3.5 Challenges to Financial Well-Being

With life expectancies increasing and the average retirement age remaining at 64 for men and 62 for women, the time period that people will spend in retirement is lengthening. It doesn't take much to understand that more assets need to be accumulated before retirement in order to cover growing retirement income needs. And, there are additional factors affecting this need for additional assets. A 2015 brief from the Center for Retirement Research stresses that in addition to increasing life expectancies, four other factors affect how adequately individuals are prepared for retirement (Munnell, 2015).

The percentage of income that Social Security is expected to replace has declined from 40% in 1985, and will continue to decline to 31% by 2030. The increasing Full Retirement Age, now 66 and it will continue to increase to 67, results in a greater reduction in Social Security benefit for those retiring before their Full Retirement Age. Also, the Medicare premium for Part B, which is automatically deducted from Social Security benefits, has been increasing and will continue to increase, reducing the monthly benefit amount paid out. As Social Security benefits have risen due to inflation more retirees are subjected to paying income taxes on up to 85% of their Social Security benefit (Munnell, 2015).

Changes to employer-sponsored retirement plans have shifted the responsibility and risk of saving for retirement from the employer to the employee. Employers have increasingly done away with traditional pension plans (defined benefit plans) that provided an income stream to retirees in retirement, and have switched to 401(k) plans. Less than half of these plans have an auto-enrollment feature, resulting in about 20% of employees not making contributions to their employer's retirement plan. The employee is responsible for choosing what to invest in within their individual retirement plan account, but often does not understand the risk associated with the investment choices available. Accumulations in these plans are

7 Planning for and Managing Costs Related to Caregiving

reduced when the participant withdraws money from the plan for various reasons before retirement.

An additional factor that jeopardizes retirement income security is rising out-of-pocket health care costs, which increase the amount of assets that need to be accumulated for retirement. Also, real interest rates have fallen since 1983 resulting in lower returns on investments that lead to lower retirement accumulations and a need to contribute greater amounts out of current income (Munnell, 2015). The Center for Retirement Research at Boston College developed the National Retirement Risk Index, which currently indicates that 52% of households are at risk for not having accumulated enough to maintain their standard of living in retirement.

Increasing numbers of the 65+ population are choosing to stay in or return to the workforce. A Stanford Center on Longevity report projects that 31% of men between the ages of 65 and 74 will be in the workforce in 2018 and 14% of men age 75+ will be working. The percentages for women in the workforce for the same age groups are 27% and 8% (Hayutin et al., 2010).

In 2014, the median income for individuals 65+ was $22,248, while the median income for 65+ households was $36,895. The sources of income for older adults include Social Security (85%), assets (63%), pensions (32%), earnings (23%), public assistance (3%), veterans' benefits (4%), and no income (1%) (Pension Rights Center, 2015). These statistics indicate that older adults are not prepared to deal with the potential costs associated with needing assistance and caregiving.

The 2013 Consumer Expenditure Survey has been analyzed to examine the relationship between age and consumer expenditures (Foster, 2015). Household income was compared to household expenditures. For households in the age 65–74 age group pre-tax income was $53,451 versus average/mean expenses of $46,757. For households in the 75+ age group pre-tax income was $34,097 compared to average/mean expenses of $34,382. Individual expense categories were calculated as a percentage of total annual expenses.

The following are the percentages for the 65–74 age group and the 75+ age group:

	65–74	75+
Food	12.9%	12.1%
Housing	33.4%	35.9%
Clothing	2.6%	2.2%
Transportation	17.0%	15.0%
Healthcare	11.1%	14.3% (These were much higher than the other age groups)
Entertainment	5.3%	4.1%
Pensions/SocSec	6.1%	2.4% (This is contributions to retirement plans and Soc. Sec. by those still working)
Other	11.5%	14.1%

In 2014, the official poverty rate was 14.8% or 46.7 million people. For the population age 65+ the rate was 10.0%, which was down 0.2% from 2013 (DeNavas, Proctor, & Proctor, 2015).

7.4 Support Systems

Developing support "systems" contributes to successful aging. Having support systems in place provides the individual and family peace of mind by knowing that plans have been made and resources identified so that the person needing assistance will be able to remain independent for as long as possible and will continue to experience a high quality of life. Support systems can take many forms, such as one individual (family member, other relative, friend, volunteer, or professional) or a team of individuals, one or more organizations (businesses, government agencies, non-profit organizations, co-operative groups, etc.), resources (such as assistive technologies), or anyone or anything that the individual may rely upon for help with any need. The types of support systems for any one individual will be unique to that individual. The purpose of support systems is to increase the individual's and/or family's quality of life, and the length of time that they can remain independent. By developing these systems now (at this point in time—whenever this is read) and reviewing them periodically, stress can be reduced and money can be saved.

7.5 Caregiving Support System

7.5.1 National Caregiving Research Report Key Findings

In 2015 the National Alliance for Caregiving (NAC) and the AARP Public Policy Institute released a lengthy research report titled, *Caregiving in the U.S. 2015* (NAC & AARP, 2015). This report contains a tremendous amount of useful information needed to understand the concept of caregiving, who is providing caregiving, and to what extent.

The following are selected key findings from this report (pp. 6–14):

- An estimated 34.2 million individuals provided unpaid care to an adult age 50 or older in the prior 12 months.
- Females represent 60% of caregivers, while males represent 40%.
- Eight out of ten caregivers provide care to one person; 85% provide care to a relative; 49% provide care to a parent or parent-in-law; 10% provide care to a spouse.
- While the average age of caregivers is 49, 7% of caregivers are 75 or older.
- On average caregivers have been providing care for 4 years; 24% have provided care for 5 years or more. Higher-hour caregivers (21 h or more) are twice as likely to have been providing care for 10 or more years.
- Sixty-five percent of care recipients are female, and average 69.4 years in age. Forty-eight percent of care recipients live in their own homes. As hours of care increase, care recipients are more likely to live with the caregiver.
- Forty-seven percent of caregivers care for someone 75 years or older.

- Fifty-nine percent of care recipients have a long-term physical condition; 35% have a short-term condition. Twenty-six percent of care recipients have a memory problem. Thirty-seven percent have more than one ongoing problem or illness.
- Main reasons given by caregivers for care recipients needing care include: old age (14%), Alzheimer's or other dementia (8%), surgery/wounds (8%), cancer (7%), mobility (7%), and mental/emotional health issues (7%).
- Caregivers spent an average of 24.4 h/week providing care, while 23% spent 41 or more h/week. Caregivers caring for a spouse spend 44.6 h/week.
- Fifty-nine percent of caregivers provided assistance with at least one Activity of Daily Living (ADL), most commonly helping the care recipient get in and out of beds or chairs (43%).
- Caregivers on average help with 4.2 out of 7 Instrumental Activities of Daily Living (IADLs), which include transportation (78%), grocery or other shopping (76%), or housework (72%).
- Caregivers also spend time interacting with various providers, agencies, and professionals on the care recipient's behalf.
- Sixty-six percent of caregivers monitor their care recipient's condition in order to adjust care, while 63% communicate with health care professionals, and 50% advocate for their care recipient.
- Fifty-seven percent of caregivers perform tasks that nurses typically perform such as injections, tube feedings, catheter and colostomy care, and other complex care responsibilities. Forty-two percent of these caregivers are doing medical/nursing tasks without any preparation. Only 14% report having received some training. Of higher-hour caregivers who are performing these kinds of tasks, 62% are doing so without prior preparation.

These are only a sampling of the key findings from this report. Additional detailed information is provided in this research report making it an extremely useful tool for anyone working with care recipients and caregivers to develop plans related to caregiving, and especially when developing a spending plan for the care recipient and for the caregiver(s) that includes expenses related to caregiving. Spending plans are one of the financial statements generated during the financial planning process.

7.5.2 Costs Associated with Caregiving

One tool that is used by financial planners when factoring in costs for long-term care in planning for retirement is the Cost of Care Survey done by Genworth. The Genworth 2015 Cost of Care Survey was used to determine some of the direct costs associated with caregiving (Genworth Life Insurance Company, 2015). This survey provides state specific data, so figures for Oklahoma are given below. Costs are provided for six types of expenses:

1. Homemaker Services: Service providing help with household tasks that cannot be managed alone. Homemaker services include "hands off" care such as cooking, cleaning, and running errands.
2. Home Health Aide Services: Home health aides offer services to people who need more extensive care. It is "hands on" personal care, but not medical care. This is the rate charged by a non-Medicare certified, licensed agency.
3. Adult Day Health Care: Provides social and support services in a community-based, protective setting. Various models are designed to offer socialization, supervision, and structured activities. Some programs may provide personal care, transportation, medical management, and meals.
4. Assisted Living Facility: Residential arrangements providing personal care and health services. The level of care is generally not as extensive as that of a nursing home, or an intermediate level of long term care.
5. Nursing Home Care: These facilities often provide a higher level of supervision and care than Assisted Living Facilities. They offer residents personal care assistance, room and board, supervision, medication, therapies and rehabilitation, and on-site nursing care 24 h a day.

The following are costs for Oklahoma:

	Minimum	Median	Maximum	Five year annual growth (%)
Homemaker Services Hourly Rates	$17	$19	$27	2
Home Health Aide Services Hourly Rates	$17	$20	$27	2
Adult Day Health Care Daily Rates	$45	$60	$75	6
Assisted Living Facility (One Bedroom–Single Occupancy) Monthly Rates	$950	$3,345	$6,430	6
Nursing Home (Semi-Private Room) Daily Rates	$110	$146	$175	2
Nursing Home (Private Room) Daily Rates	$135	$165	$340	3

The ASPE Issue Brief (Favrealt & Dey, 2015) provides useful information on the use of long-term services and supports (long-term care or LTC), the risk of needing care and the associated expenses. It estimates that about 52% of Americans turning 65 in 2015 will develop a disability serious enough to require LTC. Of the men in this group, 36.9% will need care for up to 5 years, while 39.8% of women will need care over that time. Women also surpass men in the number who will need care for 5 years or longer, 17.8% compared to 9.8%. This data is further broken down into subgroups based on income quintile at age 65, health status at age 65, and marital status at 65. Individuals in the two lowest income quintiles, whose health status is fair to poor, and who are unmarried will have the highest needs for long-term care.

This Issue Brief projects the amount of expenditures for long-term care services and supports and divides the sources of payment between Medicare, Medicaid, other public sources, out-of-pocket, and private insurance. The data is also divided into the total population using long-term care services and support and those with HIPAA-level disability. The average sum (in 2015 dollars) of LTC expenditures for both informal care and formal care from age 65 through death for adults turning 65 in 2015–2019 is predicted at $138,000. Of that total amount, Medicare may pay 9.9%, Medicaid (for those who qualify) may pay 34.3%, other public sources may pay 0.6%, out-of-pocket payments may be 52.3%, and private insurance may pay 2.7%. For individuals who are users of paid, formal LTC the total lifetime expenditure is $266,000. Payment by source percentages fall within (plus or minus) 0.3% of the percentages listed above.

This data is broken out separately for men versus women. Of note is that the percentages for Medicare payments are 11.6% for men and 9.2% for women, while the percentages for Medicaid payments are 29.2% for men and 36.8% for women. Out-of-pocket payments for men are at 55.5% versus 50.7% for women. This would indicate that women, who have longer life expectancies and make up a larger portion of the single/widowed/divorced older population, are more likely to spend the last years of their lives in nursing homes.

While $138,000 is the average expenditure for 65+ adults using both formal and informal care, the range of expenditure is broken out into categories based on spending levels at <$10,000 (5.7%), $10,000–$24,999 (3.8%), $25,000–$49,999 (5.9%), $50,000–$74,999 (5.1%), $75,000–$99,999 (4.6%), $100,000–$149,999 (6.2%), $150,000–$199,999 (3.3%), $200,000–$249,999 (2.2%), and >$250,000 (15.2%).

Important to note is that the number of individuals age 65+ who have HIPAA (Health Insurance Portability and Accountability Act) level disability (needing assistance with two out of six activities of daily living) is expected to grow from 6.3 million in 2015 to almost 15.7 million in 2065. This is the level of disability required by the majority of long-term care insurance policies for payment of benefits.

This type of information is extremely useful to financial planners when working with individuals and couples who are interested in purchasing long-term care insurance (the private insurance indicated in this Issue Brief). Choices that must be determined when purchasing long-term care insurance include the length of the benefit period (generally anywhere from 3 to 10 years; lifetime policies are difficult to find) and the amount of the daily or monthly benefit.

Information about caregiving costs paid out-of-pocket by caregivers, rather than care recipients, depends on the organization gathering the data. One annual survey, the Usage and Attitudes Survey, is conducted by Caring.com and summarized in their Senior Care Costs Index (Caring.com, September, 2014). Based on responses to the survey by individuals visiting their website, for 2014 caregiver spending broke down as follows: under $5000 (32%), $5000–$9999 (17%), $10,000–$19,999 (11%), $20,000–$29,999 (7%), $30,000–$39,999 (5%), $50,000 or more (7%) and don't know (21%). Spending on medications, personal care products, and home healthcare products ranged from less than $250 (29%) to $250–$500 (22%) to $500–$5000 (49%).

7.5.3 Indirect Costs Experienced by Employed Unpaid Caregivers

The *Caregiving in the U.S.* 2015 Report looks at data on caregivers who work (NAC & AARP, 2015). Sixty percent of caregivers were employed during the past year. Higher-hour caregivers were less likely to be employed (48%) than lower-hour caregivers (66%). Of employed caregivers, 56% worked full-time, 16% worked 30–39 h/week, and 25% worked fewer than 30 h/week. Even 21% of caregivers 65+ were employed while providing caregiving, and of those 33% worked full-time. Male caregivers were employed more often (66%) than female caregivers (55%). Hispanic (68%) and Asian (67%) caregivers were employed more often than African Americans (60%) and whites (56%).

Seventeen percent of caregivers were self-employed or owned their own business while also providing care. These caregivers reported working fewer hours than those who work for an employer (26% versus 11% of employee caregivers). They are also more likely to retire early (10% versus 3% of employee caregivers).

Caregiving impacts workers, and thus their personal finances, in a variety of ways:

- Go in late, leave early, take time off: 49%
- Leave of absence: 15%
- Reduce work hours/take a less demanding job: 14%
- Received a warning about performance/attendance: 7%
- Give up working entirely: 6%
- Turn down promotion: 5%
- Retired early: 4%
- Loss of job benefits: 3%
- Fired from job: 2%

Caregivers who work suffer financially from the above impacts in terms of loss of wages, health insurance and other job benefits, reduced retirement savings/investing, and reduced Social Security benefits. Factoring in these indirect costs related to caregiving is much more difficult to do because there is no specific formula or method for projecting what these costs may be in the future. Data that is gathered and reported is based on the past, and the resulting figures can only be used as guidelines. Estimates have been made for family caregivers who leave the workforce experiencing an average of just over $300,000 in lost wages and benefits (Feinberg & Choula, 2012). This is still important information for financial planners to have when discussing planning for caregiving with clients. While clients may wish for their spouses or adult children to provide assistance and care for them, if and when they need it, they are often unaware of the financial impact being a caregiver can have on these family members.

Another factor to consider concerning unpaid caregiving is the economic value of the services and support provided by spouses, family members, friends, and volunteers. An AARP Insight on the Issues Brief, Valuing the Invaluable: 2015 Update, states that the estimated value of unpaid contributions in 2013 was $470 billion (Reinhard, Feinberg, Choula, & Houser, 2015). Without these contributions, the costs associated with healthcare and long-term care would be considerably higher.

7.6 Implications

7.6.1 Implications for Policy: Governmental Support Related to Caregiving

With the aging population placing increasing demands on the healthcare and long-term care systems, the federal government recognizes the need to provide additional support to older Americans who require caregiving and their unpaid caregivers. The 2015 White House Conference on Aging Final Report (The White House Conference on Aging, 2015) provides an indication of the vast number of ways in which government departments and agencies are working to help individuals who need assistance with instrumental activities of daily living and activities of daily living remain independent, to help unpaid caregivers to continue to be able to assist their loved ones who need them, and to increase the numbers of paid, direct care workers that are needed and will continue to be needed to meet the demands of our aging population. One of the four common themes identified in the report as issues of significant importance to older Americans is long-term services and supports. A second theme involves efforts to encourage and support healthy aging programs with the goal being to reduce the need for long-term services and supports in order to reduce the demands being placed on governmental budgets at the federal, state, and local levels. Financial planners can support these efforts by discussing the importance of having a plan for healthy living with clients of all ages. Part of risk management involves strategies to avoid the risk if possible. Emphasizing to clients the potential for reducing both healthcare costs and caregiving costs by evaluating their current lifestyle habits and implementing a plan that includes improving nutrition, increasing physical activity, managing stress, and avoiding both tobacco and excessive alcohol consumption can help increase individual and family resilience.

Policy briefs are included in the White House Conference on Aging Final Report for each of the four common themes. Chapter II of the report lists public initiatives and private sector initiatives that have been put in place or have been proposed in each of the four areas. These are too numerous to include in this chapter. An additional resource for the benefit of caregivers that resulted from the White House Conference on Aging is titled Federal Resources for Caregivers (White House Conference on Aging, 2015). It lists resources under the U.S. Department of Health and Human Services, Administration for Community Living; the Centers for Medicare and Medicaid Services: the Center for Disease Control and Prevention; the Substance Abuse and Mental Health Services Administration; the National Institutes of Health; the HHS Office on Women's Health, The HHS Office of Disease Prevention and Health Promotion; the U.S. Department of Housing and Urban Development; the U.S. Department of Labor; the Office of Personnel Management; the Social Security Administration; and the U.S. Department of Veterans Affairs.

The Affordable Care Act (ACA), which is most well-known for the health insurance reform provisions under Title I, includes support for older Americans under Titles II – VIII (Administration on Aging, 2011). Under Title II, Role of

Public Programs, the Community First Choice Medicaid Option is established, certain barriers to providing Home and Community Based Services are removed, the Money Follows the Person Rebalancing Demonstration is extended through 2016, and funding to expand State Aging and Disability Resource Centers are among the ways older Americans are receiving assistance with caregiving needs. Title IV, Prevention of Chronic Disease and Improving Public Health, includes new initiatives focused on health promotion and disease prevention. Title V, Health Care Workforce, includes policies aimed at assuring an adequate high quality health care work force.

7.6.2 Implications for Practice

The segments of the United States and the world populations that include adults ages 65 and older are growing at an unprecedented rate. With larger numbers of older adults living longer, more of these adults are expected to have one or more chronic health conditions that will result in needing assistance with a wide variety of activities. This in turn will require larger numbers of both paid caregivers and unpaid caregivers. There is potential for demand to exceed the supply, which in economic terms indicates that both direct and indirect costs associated with caregiving will increase, and at a rate greater than that of the rate of inflation for other goods and services. The impact financially to the individual needing care, to the individuals providing care, and to the economic system as a whole is of great concern to federal and state governments. Many strategies are being developed and implemented to address these issues.

At an individual level, financial planners can help people develop plans for managing the risk that the potential cost of requiring caregiving represents. Risk management strategies include avoiding the risk as much as is possible. Emphasis is currently being placed on educating Americans about the need for healthy aging and making changes in lifestyle habits by having a healthy aging plan. Financial planners can help individuals allocate financial resources (income and assets) to achieve this goal. Along with the strategy of avoiding risk is an additional strategy to reduce the degree of the risk of financial costs related to caregiving as much as possible. An example would be evaluating the individual's living environment and determining what changes can be made to enable the individual to receive care in their own home versus in an assisted living or skilled care or memory care facility. Also, financial planners can assist people with learning about resources that are available to enable them to continue to live independently with a higher quality of life. A third strategy for managing risk is to transfer the risk to another entity such as an insurance company that provides long-term care insurance policies or to the federal and state government through the Medicaid system. More than likely, all of the above strategies will need to be employed to address the cost of caregiving for older Americans over the coming years.

Questions for Thought and Discussion

1. Talk to several relatives or friends who are older adults (age 50+) and ask each one what his or her concept of successful aging includes. How does what they think either coincide with what the discussion on successful aging in this chapter includes and/or how does their thinking differ.
2. Read one or two references cited in the section covering understanding the aging environment. Discuss what additional information you learned about the aging environment. How can you use this information in helping individuals plan for the potential for needing caregiving?
3. Often individuals will use the reasoning that the potential for needing caregiving is too far into the future and they don't want to think about it now. Suggest ways you might encourage them to begin thinking about their future today.
4. Many older adults want their adult children to care for them if and when they should need assistance. Discuss what issues you would introduce into the conversation and what pros and cons you would address.
5. Talk to someone who is currently a caregiver. Find out what they perceive are their major issues and what types of help could they use in managing the time, effort, and expenses related to caregiving.

References

Administration on Aging. (2011). Affordable Care Act: Opportunities for the aging network. Administration on Aging, Administration for Community Living, U.S. Department of Health and Human Services. Retrieved from www.aoa.gov/aging_statistics/docs/AoA_Affordable_Care.pdf

Administration on Aging. (2014). *A profile of older Americans: 2014*. Administration on Aging, Administration for Community Living, U.S. Department of Health and Human Services. Retrieved from http://www.aoa.acl.gov/aging_statistics/profile/2014/docs/2014-Profile.pdf

Caring.com. (2014, September). *Senior care cost index, 2014*. Retrieved from www.caring.com/research/senior-care-cost-index-2014

Centers for Medicare and Medicaid Services. (2014). *National health expenditures data, NHE fact sheet*. Retrieved from https://www.cms.gov/research-statistics-data-and-systems/statistics-trends-and-reports/nationalhealthexpenddata/nhe-fact-sheet.html

Centers for Disease Control and Prevention. (2013). *The state of aging and health in America 2013*. Atlanta, GA: Centers for Disease Control and Prevention, U.S. Department of Health and Human Services. Retrieved from http://www.cdc.gov/aging/pdf/state-aging-health-in-america-2013.pdf

Centers for Medicare and Medicaid Services. (2016). *Medicare and you 2016*. U.S. Government Printing Office. Retrieved from https://www.medicare.gov/Pubs/pdf/10050.pdf

Centers for Medicare and Medicaid Services. (2017). *Medicaid and CHIP, strengthening coverage, improving health*. Retrieved from https://www.medicaid.gov/medicaid/program-information/downloads/accomplishments-report.pdf

CFP Board of Standards. (2016, January). Retrieved from http://cfp.net/for-cfp-professionals/professional-standards-enforcement/compliance-resources/frequently-asked-questions/financial-planning/

DeNavas, W., Proctor, C., & Proctor, B. D. (2015). *Income and poverty in the United States: 2014*. U.S. Census Bureau. Current Population Reports, 60–252. Washington, DC: U.S. Government Printing Office. Retrieved from http://www.census.gov/content/dam/Census/library/publications/2015/demo/p60-252.pdf

Farber, N., Shinkle, D., Lynott, J., Fox-Grage, W., & Harrell, R. (2011, December). *Aging in place: A state survey of livability policies and practices*. Retrieved from http://assets.aarp.org/rgcenter/ppi/liv-com/aging-in-place-2011-full.pdf

Favrealt, M., & Dey, J. (2015). *Long-term services and supports for older Americans: Risks and financing research brief*. Washington, DC: U.S. Department of Health and Human Services. Retrieved from https://aspe.hhs.gov/sites/default/files/pdf/106211/ElderLTCrb-rev.pdf

Feinberg, L., & Choula, R. (2012, October). *Understanding the impact of family caregiving on work*. Washington, DC: AARP Public Policy Institute. Retrieved from http://www.aarp.org/content/dam/aarp/research/public_policy_institute/ltc/2012/understanding-impact-family-caregiving-work-AARP-ppi-ltc.pdf

Foster, A. C. (2015, December). *Consumer expenditures vary by age. Beyond the numbers: Prices and Spending, 4*(14). U.S. Bureau of Labor Statistics. Retrieved from http://www.bls.gov/opub/btn/volume-4/pdf/consumer-expenditures-vary-by-age.pdf

Genworth Life Insurance Company. (2015). *Genworth 2015 cost of care survey*. Retrieved from https://www.genworth.com/dam/Americas/US/PDFs/Consumer/corporate/130568_040115_gnw.pdf

Hayutin, A. M., Dietz, M., & Mitchell, L. (2010). *New realities of an older America: Challenges, changes, and questions*. Stanford Center on Longevity. Retrieved from http://longevity3.stanford.edu/wp-content/uploads/2013/01/New-Realities-of-an-Older-America.pdf

Hodes, R. J., Longo, D. L., & Ferrucci, L. (2010, July). *Healthy aging: Lessons learned from the Baltimore Longitudinal Study of Aging*. National Institute on Aging, National Institutes of Health, U.S. Department of Health and Human Services. Retrieved from https://d2cauhfh6h4x0p.cloudfront.net/s3fs-public/healthy_aging_lessons_from_the_baltimore_longitudinal_study_of_aging.pdf

Housing Commission. (2013, February). *Housing America's future: New directions for national policy*. Bipartisan Policy Center Housing Commission. Retrieved from https://cdn.bipartisanpolicy.org/wp-content/uploads/sites/default/files/BPC_Housing%20Report_web_0.pdf

Investopedia. Retrieved January, 2016, from http://www.investopedia.com/terms/f/financial_plan.asp?ad=dirN&qo=investopediaSiteSearch&qsrc=0&o=40186

Joint Center for Housing Studies of Harvard University. (2014). *Housing America's older adults: Meeting the needs of an aging population*. Retrieved from www.jchs.harvard.edu/sites/jchs.harvard.edu/files/jchs-housing_americas_older_adults_2014.pdf

Lipman, B., Lubell, J., & Salomon, E. (2012). *Housing an aging population: Are we prepared?* Center for Housing Policy. Retrieved from http://media.wix.com/ugd/19cfbe_5999f1c41ff141229f60055ad8c94e75.pdf

Lochner, K. A., Goodman, R., Posner, S., & Parekh, A. (2013). Multiple chronic conditions among Medicare beneficiaries: State level variations in prevalence, utilization, and cost, 2011. *Medicare and Medicaid Research Review, 3*(3). doi: http://dx.doi.org/10.5600/mmrr.003.03.b02.

Munnell, A. H. (2015) *Falling short: The coming retirement crisis and what to do about it*. Issue in Brief 15-7. Chestnut Hill, MA: Center for Retirement Research at Boston College. Retrieved from http://crr.bc.edu/wp-content/uploads/2015/04/IB_15-7.pdf

National Alliance for Caregiving. (2015, June). *Caregiving in the U.S. 2015*. Washington, DC: National Alliance for Caregiving and AARP Public Policy Institute. Retrieved from http://www.aarp.org/content/dam/aarp/ppi/2015/caregiving-in-the-united-states-2015-report-revised.pdf

Pension Rights Center. (2015, January). *Sources of income for older adults*. Retrieved from www.pensionrights.org/publications/statistic/sources-income-older-adults-0#ta

Quinn, J. B. (2016, January–February). How to make your money last. *AARP Bulletin/ Real Possibilities, 57*(1), 12–16.

Reinhard, S. C., Feinberg, L. F., Choula, R., & Houser, A. (2015, July). *Valuing the invaluable: 2015 update*. Insight on the issues 104. Washington, DC: AARP Public Policy Institute. Retrieved from http://www.aarp.org/content/dam/aarp/ppi/2015/valuing-the-invaluable-2015-update-new.pdf

Rowe, J. W., & Kahn, R. L. (1998). *Successful aging*. New York, NY: Dell.

Stein, M. K. (1998). *The prosperous retirement: Guide to the new reality*. Boulder, CO: EMSTCO Press.

U.S. Department of Health and Human Services. (2010). *Multiple chronic conditions—A strategic framework: Optimum health and quality of life for individuals with multiple chronic conditions*. Retrieved from http://www.hhs.gov/ash/initiatives/mcc/mcc_framework.pdf

VanDerhei, J. (2015, February). *Retirement savings shortfalls: Evidence from EBRI's Retirement Security Projection Model®*. EBRI Issue Brief no. 410. Employee Benefit Research Institute. Retrieved from https://www.ebri.org/pdf/briefspdf/EBRI_IB_410_Feb15_RS-Shrtfls.pdf

West, L. A., Cole, S., Goodkind, D., & He, W. (2014, June). *65+ in the United State: 2010, special studies*. Current Population Reports, United States Census Bureau, Department of Health and Human Services, U.S. Department of Commerce, National Institutes of Health, National Institute on Aging. Retrieved from http://www.census.gov/content/dam/Census/library/publications/2014/demo/p23-212.pdf

White House Conference on Aging. (2015). *White House Conference on Aging: Final Report*. Retrieved from www.whitehouseconferenceonaging.gov/2015-whcoa-final-report.pdf

Index

A
Actigraphy, 69
Activities of daily living (ADLs), 9, 31
Administration on aging, 126
Adult Day Health Care, 134
The Affordable Care Act, 137
Agency thinking, 84
Aging environment, 125–131
Aging population, 137
Alzheimer's disease, 101
Antioxidants, 54
Area Agency on Aging (AAA), 34
Arthritis (osteoarthritis/rheumatoid), 53
Assistant Secretary for Planning and Evaluation (ASPE), 121, 134
Assisted living facility, 134
Atherosclerosis, 54
Atrophic gastritis, 49

B
Baby boom generation, 125
Baltimore Longitudinal Study of Aging, 128
Bipartisan Policy Center Housing Commission, 128
Bone fractures, 53

C
Calcium, 53
Calories, 47, 48
Canadian Institute for Health Information (CIHI), 104
Canadian provinces, 104
Carbohydrate, 48
Caregiver family therapy (CFT)
 age-related problems, 35
 care structure, 37, 38
 components, 36
 definition, 35
 naming the problem, 36, 37
 role reverberations, 39
 role structure, 38
 self-care, 39, 40
 widening the lens, 40, 41
Caregiver resilience
 CDC, 65
 evidenced-based design, 64
 furniture, 65, 67
 guidelines, 73
 health and wellbeing, 74
 hospital settings, 65
 implications for practice, 72–73
 knees and ankles, 72
 rationale, 68
 rural area hospital, 68
 seat
  angle, 73
  depth, 73
  height, 73
  width, 73
 Sit2Sleep, 65, 67, 69
 sitting and sleeping, 73
 usability test, 65
 venous blood flow, 69
 Venous Chair, 64
 working hypothesis, 68

Index

Caregivers, 58
  burden, 109–110
  implications
    older care recipient's resilience, 54, 55
Caregiving burden and stress, 81
Caregiving families, 28–30, 35–41
  CFT (*see* Caregiver family therapy (CFT))
  characteristic, family life, 27
  child-rearing, 27
  chronic diseases, 28
  family care trajectories, 31, 32
  family resilience processes, 28
  healthcare systems, 28
  help-seeking, 32, 33
  interventions, 34, 35
  life expectancy, 27
  social location
    caregiver assumption, 29
    chronic disease, 29
    cultural contexts, 29
    electronic record systems, 29
    fragmented health systems, 28
    human life and quality of life, 29
    mental health services, 29
    models, 29, 30
    outpatient/inpatient care systems, 29
    self-management, 29
  stages, 32
Caregiving in the U.S. 2015, 132
Caregiving support system, 132, 133
The Center for Disease Control (CDC), 64–65
Center for Housing Policy, 127
Centers for Medicare and Medicaid
    Services, 128
Certified Financial Planner (CFP) Board of
    Standards, 122
Chronic conditions, 129
Complementary caregiving, 18
Conjoint caregiving, 18
Consumer Expenditure Survey, 131
Cost of Care Survey, 133
Cushioning, 73

D
Dehydration, 51
Dementia, 2–4, 21, 99, 107
Department of Health and Human Services,
    128, 129
Department of Health and Wellness (DHW), 104
Depression, 50
Dietary calcium intake, 53
Dietary fiber, 48
2015–2020 Dietary Guidelines for Americans, 56

Dietary Reference Intake (DRI), 48
Dietary supplements, 56

F
2010 Facility Guideline Institute's *Guidelines
    for Design and Construction of
    Health Care Facilities* (FGI), 65
Family adaptive systems (FAS)
  application, 13–15
  control systems, 17–19
  emotion systems, 19
  FSRS, 19, 20
  maintenance systems, 16
  meaning systems, 17
  short- and long- term adaptation, 16
  stress response system, 16
Family caregiver perspectives
  ability, 115
  anger and guilt, 112–113
  behavioral and psychological
    symptoms, 101
  Canadian provinces, 104, 117
  caregiver resilience, 100–101
  care recipient, 115
  care transitions, 102–103
  continuum of care, 102
  data analysis, 108–109
  dementia, 114
  DHW, 113, 115
  environmental stressors, 100
  factors, 100
  implications, 115–118
  individuals, 102
  interviews, 106
  LTC, 99, 101, 116
  on/off conceptualization, 116
  participants, 113
  policy makers, 116
  practice, 103
  principle, 102
  transitional care, 112
Family caregiving, 5
  care recipient, 1
  FRM (*see* Family resilience model (FRM))
  medical and social services, 1
  well-being, 1
Family control systems, 17–19
Family emotion systems, 19
Family-home health care system, 20
Family maintenance systems, 16
Family meaning systems, 17
  identity, 17
  meaning making, 17

worldview
    collective approach, 17
    frameability, 17
    relativism, 17
    shared purpose, 17
    spirituality, 17
Family resilience model (FRM), 7–24, 74, 93
    adaptation
        adequate functioning, 10
        adult child/grandchild, 10
        bonadaptation (positive adaptation), 9
        dementia, 10
        family adaptive systems, 11
        family situational meanings, 11–16
        family subsystems, 10
        health stressors, 11
        maladaptation (negative family adaptation), 10
        medical/social services, 9
        proximal care systems, 9
        short- and long- term, 9
        steeling effect, 9
    core resilience concepts, 7
    dementia, 24
    distal and proximal ecosystems, 6, 20
    family system levels, 24
    FAS (*see* Family adaptive systems (FAS))
    implications
        Alzheimer's diagnosis, 21
        dementia, 21
        emotion system, 22
        familiso and *respecto*, 22
        family caregiving, 23
        family stress response system, 22
        genogram, Alvarez family, 22
        intellectual and developmental disabilities, 21, 23
        maintenance and meaning systems, 22
        marital satisfaction, 21
        meaning and control systems, 22
        multiple family system levels, 21
        principles, policymakers and practitioners, 23, 24
        proximal-ecosystem (healthcare and social services), 22
    modifications, 5, 6
    multiple family systems levels, 5
    protection and vulnerabilities
        caregiver self-efficacy, 9
        caregiving stressors, 8
        family-proximal (close) ecosystem, 8
        financial management, 9
        medical and social services communities, 8
        on-going interaction patterns, 8
        promotive and protective processes, 8
        vertical/horizontal stressors, 8
    proximal ecosystems, 6
    significant risk
        degenerative health conditions, 7
        family systems, 7
        specific family stressors, 7
        status risk, 7
Family stress response system (FSRS), 19, 20
Fats, 49
Fiduciary duty, 123
Financial planning process, 121, 123
Financial planning subject areas, 123
Full Retirement Age, 130

H

Home health aide services, 134
Homemaker services, 134
Hope
    agency and pathways, 84, 85
    apathy, 87
    and caregiving, 89
    caregivers, 81, 84
    depression scores, 89
    despair, 87
    hospitalization, 82
    human behavior, 83
    individuals, 84
    mental energy, 84
    NAC/AARP, 81
    positive psychology, 82
    post-traumatic stress, 89
    practice and policy, 93
    protective factors, 89
    resilience, 89–93
    self-efficacy, 85
    social well-being, 85
    stress, 82
    theory, 83, 84
    viable pathways, 88
Horizontal stressors, 7, 8
Human adaptive systems, 16

I

Insight into the Determinants of Exceptional Aging and Longevity (IDEAL), 128
Institutionalization, 110
Instrumental activities of daily living (IADLs), 9, 31
Intervention designs, 70–72
Issue Brief projects, 135

J
Joint Center for Housing Studies of Harvard University, 127

K
401(k) plans, 130

L
Living arrangements, 127–128
Long term care (LTC), 99

M
Mindfulness-based stress reduction, 41
Minerals, 49
MyPlate Daily Checklist, 56

N
National Institute on Aging's Baltimore Longitudinal Study of Aging, 125
National Retirement Risk Index, 131
Nursing Home Care, 134

O
Older adults' nutritional needs
　calories, 47, 48
　carbohydrate, 48
　fats, 49
　fiber, 48
　good nutrition, 58
　protein, 48
　vitamins and minerals, 49
　water, 49
Older care recipients' food intake
　appetite, 50, 51
　chewing and swallowing, 51
　cognition function, 53, 54
　energy, strength, coordination and range of motion, 52, 53
　thirst, 51
Optimism theory, 85, 86

P
Parental caregiving, 89
Patented Probax cushion design, 67
Pathway thinking, 84
Patient-reported satisfaction, 68
Periodontal disease, 51
Positive psychology, 82–83
Premium, 129

ProBax, 64
Prosperous retirement, 125
Protein, 48

Q
Qualitative observations, 107

R
Racial and ethnic diversity, 126
Resilience processes, 90
Ridgemont Continuing Care Center, 105
Ridgemont resident, 109

S
Self-efficacy, 85
Seligman's optimism theory, 86
Senior Care Costs Index, 135
Single entry access system, 105, 111
Sit2Sleep design, 70, 76–78
Sleep efficiency, 69
Social security, 130
Sound locking mechanism, 71
Stonebridge resident, 110
Substance Abuse and Mental Health Services Administration, 35
Substitutive caregiving, 18

T
Tooth decay, 51

U
Unexpected career of caregiver, 99
Unintentional weight loss, 48
U.S. Department of Agriculture (USDA), 48
U.S. Department of Health and Human Services (USDHHS), 48, 126

V
Venous Chair, 64, 66, 69, 75, 76
Venous stasis, 66
Vertical stressors, 8
Vitamins, 49, 53

W
Water, 49
White House Conference on Aging Final Report, 137

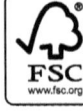

If you have any concerns about our products,
you can contact us on
ProductSafety@springernature.com

In case Publisher is established outside the EU,
the EU authorized representative is:
**Springer Nature Customer Service Center GmbH
Europaplatz 3, 69115 Heidelberg, Germany**

Printed by Libri Plureos GmbH
in Hamburg, Germany

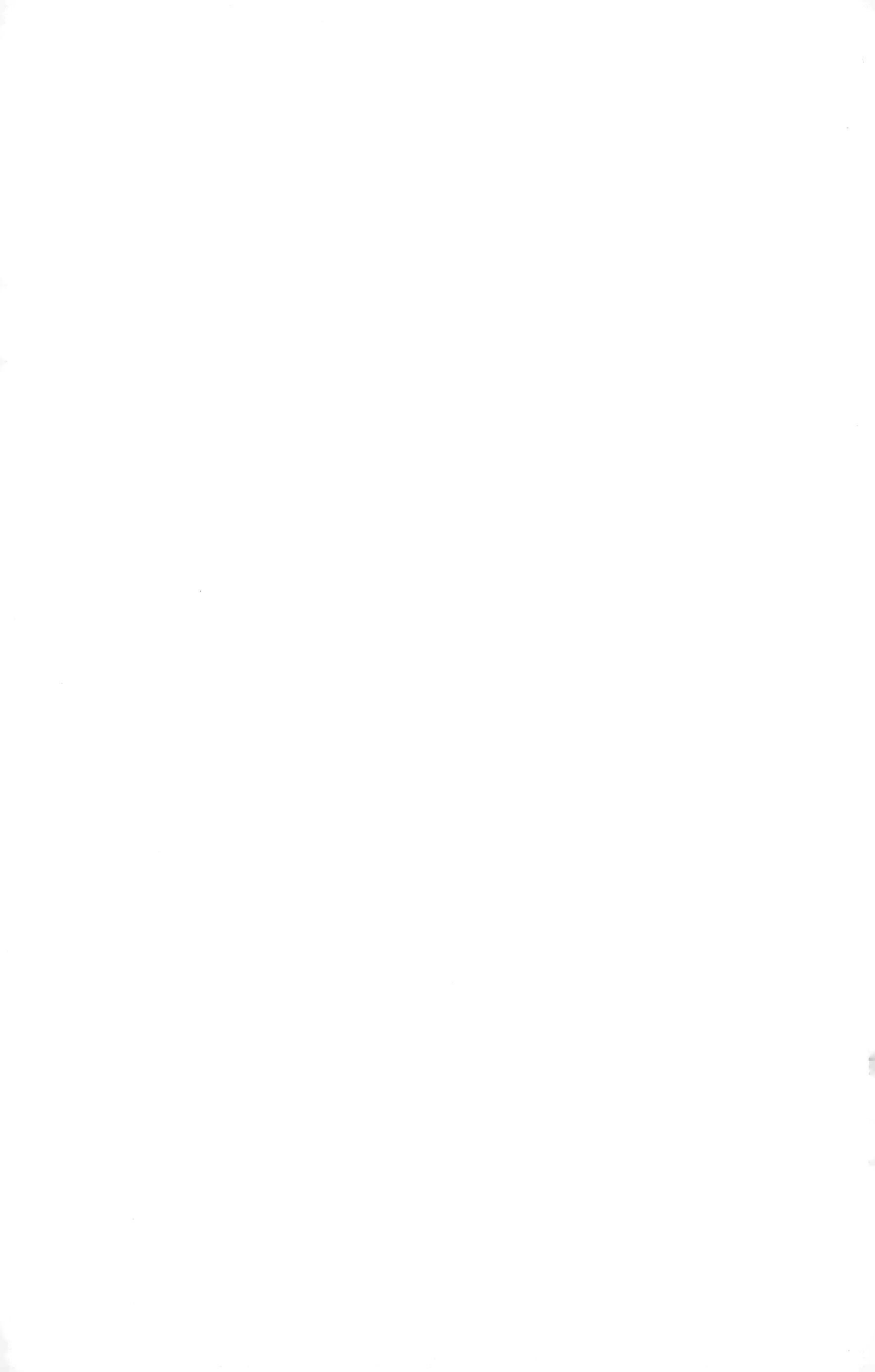